KUNDALINI YOGA

Skyhorse Publishing books may be purchased in bulk at special discounts for sales promotion, corporate gifts, fund-raising, or educational purposes. Special editions can also be created to specifications. For details, contact the Special Sales Department, Skyhorse Publishing, 307 West 36th Street, 11th Floor, New York, NY 10018 or info@skyhorsepublishing.com.

Skyhorse® and Skyhorse Publishing® are registered trademarks of Skyhorse Publishing, Inc.®, a Delaware corporation.

Visit our website at www.skyhorsepublishing.com.

10 9 8 7 6 5 4 3 2 1

Library of Congress Cataloging-in-Publication Data is available on file.

Cover photo credit Brigitte Sporrer

Print ISBN: 978-1-63220-685-5
Ebook ISBN: 978-1-62087-552-0

Printed in China

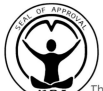

This publication has received the KRI Seal of Approval. This Seal is given only to products that have been reviewed for accuracy and integrity of the sections containing the 3HO lifestyle and Kundalini Yoga as taught by Yogi Bhajan.

KUNDALINI YOGA

– Techniques for Developing Strength, Awareness, and Character –

ATHANASIOS KARTA SINGH MEGARISIOTIS
PHOTOGRAPHS BY BRIGITTE SPORRER

Translation by Tobi Haberstroh

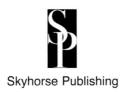

Skyhorse Publishing

CONTENTS

"HAPPINESS IS YOUR BIRTHRIGHT." —Y. B.

FOREWORD

Yoga is a philosophical teaching that originated in India. It encompasses a holistic system of practices, which are meant to bring the body, mind, and soul in tune.

KUNDALINI YOGA is a comprehensive path of growth and life that demands neither asceticism nor seclusion. It is much more about linking together the spiritual practice and the everyday life of those who practice it.

For millennia, KUNDALINI YOGA remained a well-guarded secret of great Yogis. In 1968, Yogi Bhajan revealed these secret teachings to the Western world. This Yoga of awareness makes it possible to come to understand and live the different levels of being through body- and energy-work that is harmonizing and calming. The results can be felt after just a short time. In comparison with other Yoga paths, the exercises in KUNDALINI YOGA tend to be more active and dynamic but do not include extreme stretches or postures. Therefore, KUNDALINI YOGA can be learned and practiced by everyone.

This book offers the opportunity to learn the basic principles of KUNDALINI YOGA step by step. It explains the most popular seated positions, breath techniques, hand positions, and the most commonly used poses. These instructions prepare you for the main chapter, *Kriyas*. Kriyas are exercise series that combine all the elements of the Yoga practice and have a specific result on the body, mind, and soul. The end of each routine is meditation.

I wish every beginner, and every Yogini and Yogi, much happiness with this book!

Light and Love,
Athanasios Karta Singh

"Just as all rivers end up in the ocean, all forms of Yoga end up raising the Kundalini. Kundalini is the creative potential of every human being." —Y. B.

KUNDALINI YOGA
YOGA OF AWARENESS
KUNDAL: THE CURL IN A LOCK OF HAIR OF THE BELOVED

KUNDALINI YOGA is regarded as the most comprehensive and extensive of all Yoga methods. In contrast to the other traditional Yoga teachings, which deepen partial aspects of classical Yoga, all the original elements are inseparably connected in KUNDALINI YOGA.

KUNDALINI YOGA is not dogmatic and demands neither asceticism nor seclusion. In contrast, it can be integrated directly into your daily life.

KUNDALINI YOGA attempts to unite body, mind, and soul through exercises, meditation, and breathing exercises. This comprehensive Yoga philosophy teaches a yogic diet and lifestyle. In addition, it includes the healing technique **Sat Nam Rasayan,** the martial art **Gatka,** white **Tantric Yoga,** and Yoga for pregnancy.

It is the highest goal of KUNDALINI YOGA to balance the duality in people. This occurs through the unification of *Shakti* and *Shiva.* According to tantric teachings (tantric = unifying, interweaving), Shakti, the female creative force, rests at the base of the spine and is the living, constantly changing energy. Located at the crown of the head is Shiva, the consciousness, the male, unchanging, observing energy. These two poles unite through the awakening of the Kundalini. That serpentine energy, which sleeps at the base of the spine in three and a half coils, is the infinite life energy in every human being. It is necessary to awaken it and let it ascend along the spine to the crown of the head through each energy center.

To make dormant Kundalini energy flow, KUNDALINI YOGA works with movement and dynamics combined with breath work and sounds. Each practice series relates to a specific area of the body, mind, and soul. Through the systematic adjustment of the length and sequence of particular elements, each series has a harmonizing and healthy physical and mental effect.

Many exercises promote blood flow and toning of certain muscle groups and improve posture. The lymphatic and glandular systems are stimulated; the organs are massaged and strengthened in their respective functions. Circulation is regulated, and the strengthened energy in the meridians begins to flow. Holistic bodily well-being arises.

KUNDALINI YOGA works on various mental levels. First and foremost comes the awareness that personal happiness can be learned and controlled. Old thought and behavior patterns transform so that the desired changes can replace them. Personal responsibility, intuition, and perception emerge.

KUNDALINI YOGA is the Yoga of awareness. It strengthens the ability to recognize and clear away the causes of negative emotions. It intensifies the perception of inner desires and needs and allows you to live your truth with attentiveness and concentration.

YOGA
YUI = BINDING TOGETHER, BRACING, HARNESSING, YOKING
YUGI = YOKE, HARNESS

The teachings of Yoga originated in India. Yoga attempts to unite body, mind, and soul and thus to develop the entire human potential. This is accomplished through the interaction of physical poses, breath work, and meditation.

'Yoga' means unification and integration but at the same time can be understood as harnessing or yoking the body to the soul. In this sense, the material body represents the wagon and the soul represents the traveler.

Yoga is a millennia-old science. Its development was first set down in writing some 2,500 years ago. The most important of these Yoga texts are the
* *Upanishads,* which pertain to Gyan Yoga,
* *Bhagavad Gita,* which includes all Yoga paths but concentrates on Karma Yoga and Bhakti Yoga,
* *Hatha Yoga Pradipika,* which defines Hatha Yoga,
* *Yoga Sutras,* which describes the royal discipline of Raya Yoga.

YOGA-SUTRA
SUTRA = THREAD, CORD

The Indian philosopher Patanjali (who probably lived in the second century B.C.E.) wrote *Yoga Sutras,* which has been completely preserved. However, it is believed that in the following centuries, many parts were added to this oldest Yoga text. The *Yoga Sutras* consists of 195 short verses and describes the essence of the Yoga path in a concentrated form. In it, Patanjali describes the *ashtanga.* These are the elements of the eight-fold path of Yoga, which build upon each other and form an indivisible whole:

1	Yama	Morality, ethics, abstinence, self-control
2	Niyama	Self-discipline, rules of conduct
3	Asana	Control of the body through poses
4	Pranayama	Control of the breath through breathing exercises
5	Pratyahara	Control of the senses
6	Dharana	Concentration
7	Dhyana	Meditation
8	Samadhi	Immersion, enlightenment, actualization of the Higher Self

THE YOGA PATHS OF THE CLASSICAL INDIAN TEACHINGS

GYAN (JNANA) YOGA – YOGA OF KNOWLEDGE

Gyan Yoga is concerned exclusively with understanding the Yoga path. The study should cause consciousness of all deeds, feelings, and thoughts and awareness of the principle of karma and reincarnation. This knowledge should lead to the manifestation of the Higher Self and enable deliverance from the cycle of reincarnation.

KARMA YOGA – YOGA OF SELFLESS SERVICE

Karma Yoga is about using up existing karma without building any new. This is made possible through selfless actions, which lead finally to the dissolution of the ego. In Karma Yoga, the same energetic processes are activated as those in KUNDALINI YOGA that allow the awakening of Kundalini.

BHAKTI YOGA – YOGA OF DEVOTION

Bhakti Yoga is the path to unity with the infinite, with the Creator and the Creation, through universal and unconditional love, meditation, devotion, and self-sacrifice.

HATHA YOGA – YOGA OF BODY AWARENESS

This is the most popular form of Yoga in the Western world. It produces a balance between the positive, solar (= ha) and the negative, lunar (= tha) polarities. *Hatha* means the effort necessary to achieve the ultimate goal of Yoga. Hatha Yoga is rather physically focused, and it was first employed in support of other forms of Yoga because of the strengthening and mobilizing effects of the exercises. However, it was developed further and described for the first time in the *Hatha Yoga Pradipika* as an independent form of Yoga. The physical aspect of Hatha Yoga is an essential prerequisite to reaching the higher levels of Raya Yoga.

RAYA YOGA – THE ROYAL MASTERY OF THE MIND

The royal Yoga concentrates on the meditative level of Yoga. Visualization, attentiveness, introspection of the mind, and meditation on the chakras produce control of the mental body and the thoughts. KUNDALINI YOGA is a Raya Yoga.

PRANA AND APANA
PRANA = SPIRIT, BREATH OF LIFE, LIFE FORCE, ENERGY, AIR

Prana is the universal life energy, which permeates every living body. This positively charged sun energy is active above the navel and has a vitalizing and warming effect on the body.

One part of prana is *apana,* the eliminating energy. This moon energy, which is active below the navel, regulates the body's elimination processes and pushes away negative energy. Apana cleanses, calms, cools, and regenerates body and mind.

NADI
NADI = CHANNEL, CONDUIT

72,000 nadis are described in the old Yoga texts. These are subtle energy channels which supply the body with prana. There are three main energy channels of particular importance: sushmana, ida, and pingala. These three nadis flow through all chakras and spring from the root chakra, the resting place of the Kundalini energy.

SUSHMANA   The central channel, which runs along the spinal column and ends at the crown chakra. Kundalini energy flows through sushmana.

IDA   Runs left of sushmana from the root chakra to the left nostril. Apana flows through ida.

PINGALA   Runs right of sushmana from the root chakra to the right nostril. Prana flows through pingala.

KUNDALINI AWAKENING

When you hold an exhale, prana flows from the upper chakras to the center of the body, to the navel chakra. With a subsequent held exhale, apana rises from the lower chakras to the navel chakra. From this meeting and uniting of both energies in the center of the body comes the so-called *white heat.* It sinks through the sushmana down to the root chakra, where the Kundalini energy awakens. Breath control and power of will allow the Kundalini to rise higher and to come to the higher-seated chakras slowly and continuously. In this manner, lower energies can be dispelled or transformed into higher energies. It is important to cleanse the nadis of blockages and impurities using breath control (pranayama), exercises (asanas), and the engaging of body locks (bandhas) to allow the free flow of Kundalini.

SIRI SINGH SAHIB BHAI SAHIB HARBHAJAN SINGH KHALSA YOGIJI
YOGI BHAJAN

Yogi Bhajan was born August 26, 1929, as the son of a doctor in Kot Harkam in present-day Pakistan (then India). He began his study of Yoga as a child and at 16 was affirmed as a master of KUNDALINI YOGA by Sant Hazara Singh. During countless periods of study with various spiritual teachers in different ashrams, he acquainted himself with natural healing and Vedic philosophy. At the same time, he completed a degree in economics at the University of Punjab. He married in the Sikh tradition, started a family, and was a successful Indian civil servant.

In 1968 Yogi Bhajan was invited to Canada to give a lecture on Yoga. With this he broke the tradition of only passing on the secret, millennia-old KUNDALINI YOGA teachings orally to a few select students. He began to spread these teachings openly. Until his death, he passed on not only body and meditation exercises but also taught healing techniques like Sat Nam Rasayan, yogic massage, the martial art Gatka, as well as the entire yogic lifestyle.

After he moved to Los Angeles in 1969, Yogi Bhajan founded the nonprofit organization *3HO* (Happy, Healthy, Holy Organization). The concern of this foundation is to spread KUNDALINI YOGA, meditation and humanistic sciences with the goal of improving people's physical wellness and supporting spiritual growth. The three principles of the organization—living healthily, happily, and holistically—correspond to the yogic philosophy of uniting body, mind, and soul. In 1994 the 3HO became a member of the NGO (Non-Governmental Organization) of the United Nations and is represented there by Yogi Bhajan's wife, Dr. Bibiji Inderjit Kaur.

Yogi Bhajan was not only a master of KUNDALINI YOGA but also a successful businessman and the founder of various peace and human-rights organizations. He always called on his students to seek their place in the world and be successful. He particularly encouraged women to take on leadership positions in public life. As a doctor of communication studies, he taught how to develop conscious and purposeful communication skills.

On October 6, 2004, Yogi Bhajan died in Española, New Mexico. He was posthumously awarded the Heart of Humanity Award for lifetime achievement for his extraordinary contributions to world peace, social responsibility, and the advancement of the human mind.

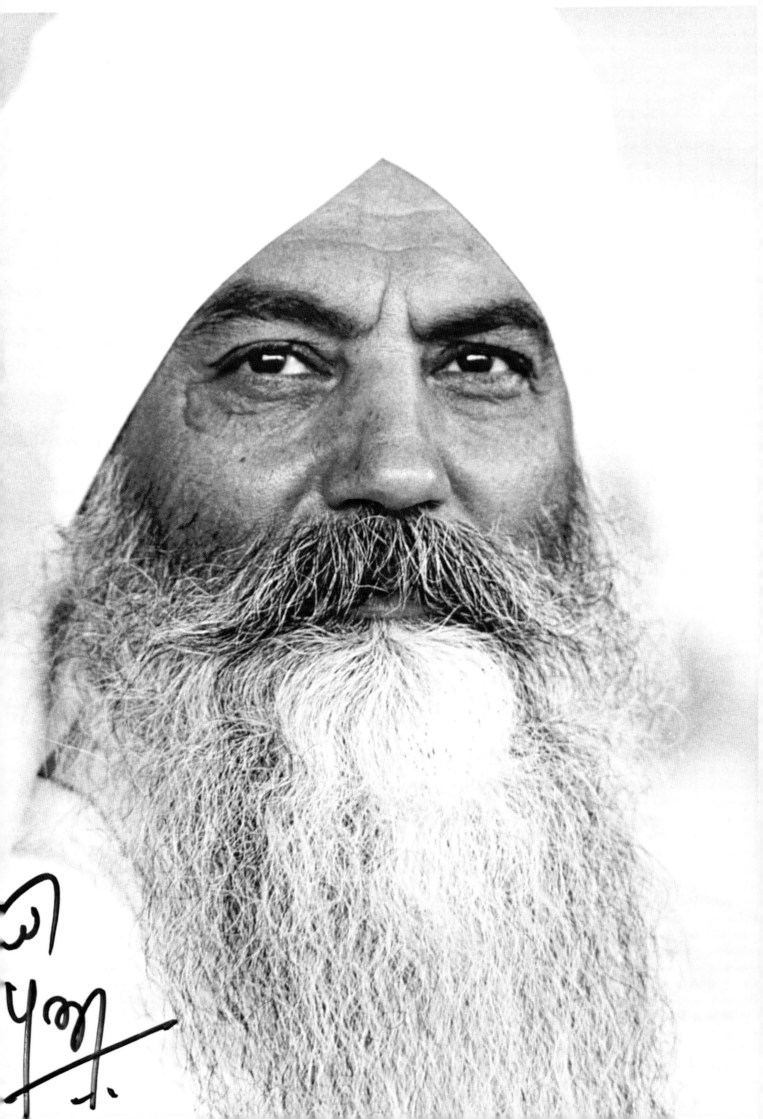

"The first thing that you must learn to understand as a human being is the instrument of your movement—the physical body. All these systems (glandular system, circulatory system, respiratory sytem, heartbeat, brain, and nervous system) are connected with one another via a structure of flesh and bones. It is a functionally cohesive system. And as such, it needs attention, care, and fine-tuning." —Y. B.

SUGGESTIONS FOR YOUR PRACTICE

Yoga is not gymnastics or a competition. The goal is not to achieve an outwardly perfect form through excessive ambition but rather to experience your own spirituality and the interaction of body and mind in each pose.

- Perform the asanas on a soft, not too cold surface such as a mat made of natural materials. A sheepskin has the benefit of having a good insulating effect.

- Clothing should be comfortable, not too tight, and preferably made of natural materials.

- You should be barefoot so that the nerve endings in your feet can connect with outside energies.

- If possible, wear a head covering. This helps to better guide and preserve energy.

- For two hours before Yoga, you should not eat anything heavy, at most some fruit. However, drink as much water as possible before, during, and after a Yoga session.

- Keep your eyes closed during all exercises so that you can concentrate better on the third eye and will be less distracted by outside influences.

- Always breathe through the nose unless otherwise specified in the instructions.

- As a beginner, you can shorten the recommended times proportionally for all exercises (for example, from 4-2-2 minutes to 2-1-1 minutes), include additional resting phases, or replace difficult exercises with simpler variations.

- Do not overstrain yourself with the exercises, and only take the poses as far as your physical condition allows.

- In the case of spinal problems, practice the simpler variation of the exercise, decrease the recommended time, or run through the exercise mentally.

- In the case of acute pain, end the exercise immediately and assume a relaxed pose.

- In the case of health problems, always consult a doctor first to avoid potential injury.

- During menstruation and pregnancy, do not practice the breath of fire, inversions, or exercises which exert pressure on the abdominal cavity.

A KUNDALINI YOGA session is divided into the following sections:

1	Attunement	Sit upright and sing the Adi mantra 3 times.
2	Kriya	Choose the kriya that speaks to you most at the moment and practice the exercise in the given sequence.
3	Deep Relaxation	Relax in a supine position.
4	Meditation	Find a meditation that fits with the kriya and your current situation.
5	Ending Chant	End your Yoga practice by singing "May the Long Time Sun" and by singing the mantra SAT NAM three times.

To mobilize the spine in all directions and to prepare the hip and seat musculature, you can do some additional warm-up exercises before the attunement. These should be easy and should not involve any intense bending or stretching; otherwise, they could energetically influence the effects of the following kriya. Suitable asanas are camel ride, Sufi circles, cat-cow, and torso twists.

"You must transform and transcend your unconscious habit of pitying yourself and having feelings of inferiority if you want to grow and feel the experience of your mind reaching into infinity." —Y. B.

SEATED POSES

In the *Yoga Sutras* of Patanjali, the only asana mentioned is a seated position with crossed legs. This seated pose is stable and comfortable and thus lends itself very well to deep meditation.

In KUNDALINI YOGA, there is a multitude of seated asanas. There are many variations to choose from based on physical condition and skill level.

It is very important to hold the spine straight no matter which seated pose is chosen. The crown of the head is always located directly above the tailbone, creating a line with it. The navel point is gently pulled in toward the spinal column and the chest gently lifted. The shoulders relax down and are pulled back gently. By engaging the throat lock, the neck is elongated and the crown becomes the highest point of the body.

The energies awakened in the asanas and meditation can only unfurl and transform in an erect spinal column. Any compression or bending of the back holds the risk of an energy blockage or an undesired transformation of the energy.

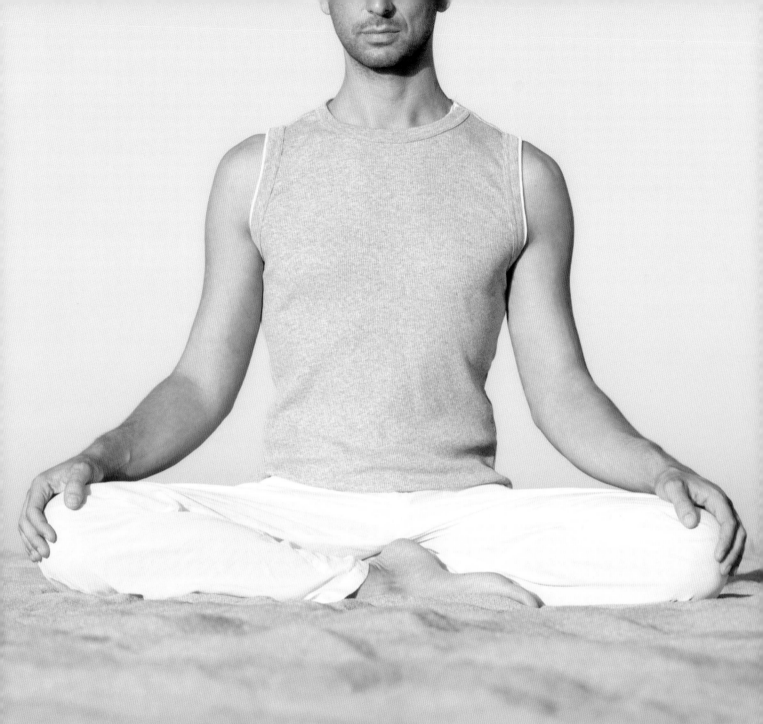

SIMPLE SEATED POSE
MUKTASANA

Sit up straight and cross your legs. Ideally you should lay one heel as close as possible to your body and the other heel directly in front of it, so that the feet lie at the center of your body. Let the knees relax and sink as far as possible toward the floor. Take care that your spine is straight from your coccyx to the crown of your head. Tilt your pelvis slightly forward to prevent curving the back. If it is difficult to sit up straight, you can sit on a pillow or a folded blanket. Switch the positions of your legs from time to time to avoid applying uneven force.

If you have less experience, you can instead sit in the tailor pose (sukhasana).

The simple seated pose is the most used seated asana in KUNDALINI YOGA. It allows for a stable and straight posture and requires less flexibility of the pelvis and legs than the lotus position.

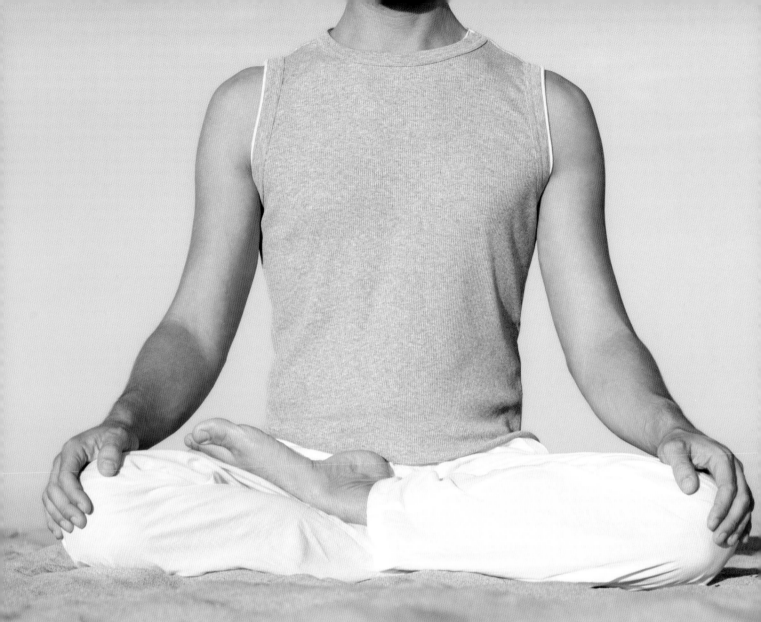

HALF LOTUS
ARDHA PADMASANA

Sit up straight in the simple seated pose with your left heel lying close to you. Lay the right foot on the left thigh and turn it gently, so that the sole of your foot faces upward and the knee sinks to the floor, relaxed. Switch the positions of your legs from time to time to avoid applying uneven force.

The half lotus requires more flexibility of the pelvis and legs than the simple seated pose and is the simplified version of the complete lotus pose.

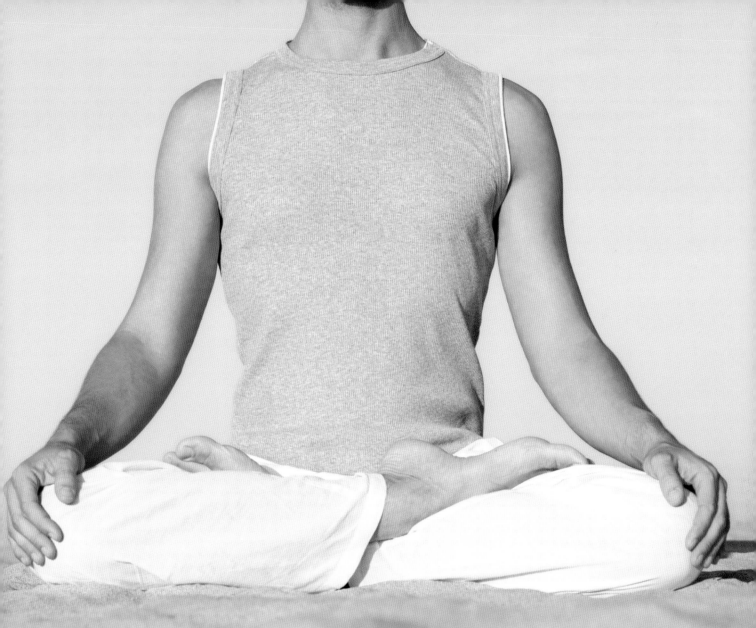

LOTUS
PADMASANA

From the simple seated pose, lay the right foot on the left thigh and the left foot on the right thigh. Relax the feet; the soles of the feet face upward. The knees touch the floor. Make sure to keep a straight posture while in the lotus position. The chin is drawn in and the shoulders are relaxed. Switch the positions of your legs from time to time to avoid applying uneven force.

This classic Yoga pose requires regular practice and a high degree of flexibility in the pelvic area. Because the lotus allows for long, still sitting, it lends itself particularly to deep meditation. Keeping the erect spine stable and firm can prevent back pain.

KNEELING POSE
VAJRASANA

Come into a kneeling position with your knees and your heels touching. The tops of your feet lie flat on the floor. Sit with your sitz bones on your heels. Make sure that your back is straight and your shoulders are relaxed. Hold your pelvis straight so that you do not hollow your lower back. If you have less experience, you can also place a pillow or a rolled-up blanket under your feet or between your heels and sitz bones.

You can choose the kneeling pose as an alternative if the seated position with crossed legs is difficult for you.

CELIBATE POSE

Come into the kneeling pose. Spread your feet slightly wider than your hips. The knees stay together. Turn the feet slightly in toward the axis of your body. Let the sitz bones slowly sink between your legs to the floor. The heels and hip bones should remain about a finger's width apart. Straighten up your spine and relax your shoulders. Make sure that your weight is evenly distributed between both sitz bones.
If you have difficulties with this pose, you can make it easier by laying a pillow or rolled-up blanket under your seat.

"You live through your breath, you are a product of your breath, and the realization of your goals occurs through your breath. In the moment that you are truly united with your breath, the universe streams into you." —Y. B.

PRANAYAMA
PRANA = LIFE ENERGY; YAMA = CONTROL

Pranayama is a fundamental element of KUNDALINI YOGA and, translated simply, means: control or guidance of the breath.

Breath provides the organism with oxygen and enriches body and mind with prana. The goal of many breathing exercises in Yoga is awareness and attentiveness regarding the breath.

Pranayama techniques make it possible to influence the physical and mental planes through the interaction of rhythm, form, and depth of the breath. The fewer breaths you take (optimally four to eight in a minute) the greater your relaxation, concentration, and inner clarity. This calms the nervous system and supports healing processes.

In addition to the *long deep breath,* other breath techniques will be used in the KUNDALINI YOGA exercises and meditations. Among others, the *breath of fire,* the *left and right nostril breath,* or the *cooling breath through a rolled tongue* will be utilized to achieve various results.

In many exercises and meditations it is necessary to hold the breath intentionally for a while. This can be done at different points in the breath cycle: after the inhale or after the exhale. In this book, holding your breath after inhaling is indicated simply with the phrase *holding the inhale. Holding the exhale,* on the other hand, means that the breath should be held after exhaling. This difference is vital and the instructions should always be followed.

LONG DEEP BREATH
YOGIC BREATH

The long deep breath is divided into three phases with about five to eight breaths per minute. It begins and ends in the stomach.

Sit in the simple seated pose with a straight back, engage the throat lock, and concentrate on your third eye. Begin to inhale slowly and deeply. Breathe first into the stomach, so that the relaxed stomach muscles come forward and the diaphragm is pulled downward. The next step is to breathe into the chest. The ribcage expands, the ribs come forward and are gently pulled apart. Breathe in further, so deeply that the upper ribcage, sternum, and collarbone are lifted upward. Hold your breath for a moment and then exhale long and deep in the reverse order. First the collarbone and upper ribcage sink, then the central ribcage. Finally the abdominal wall also sinks and pushes the remaining breath out of the body. In your mind, let the mantra SAT resonate with each inhale and the mantra NAM resonate with each exhale. Make sure that you only breathe through your nose and that you inhale and exhale completely with each breath.

As opposed to the energetic breath of fire, the long deep breath has a calming, centering, and relaxing effect. It harmonizes and relaxes the internal organs, activates glandular function, increases lung volume and raises oxygen transfer. At the same time, pulse and blood pressure are reduced, body pH is regulated, and the self-cleaning mechanisms of the blood and metabolism are activated. In this manner, the self-healing processes of the body and mind are promoted. The aura is positively charged and provides physical and psychic protection from negative outside influences. The long deep breath promotes health and vitality and strengthens the stamina of your body and mind, as well as your concentration and awareness of your connection with the universe.

BREATH OF FIRE
AGNI PRANA

With the breath of fire—without pausing between inhaling and exhaling—
about two to three breaths are taken in a second.

Take a relaxed, seated pose and concentrate on your navel point. Begin fire breathing, breathing quickly
through the nose into the belly. The relaxed abdominal wall curves forward slightly; the diaphragm is pulled
downward. When you exhale, pull the stomach and diaphragm in quickly towards the spine, pushing the
breath out through the nose. The throat lock should be engaged during the whole exercise. Make sure
that your inhales and exhales are the same length and strength. During the breath of fire, only activate
the stomach muscles and deliberately relax the initial tension in legs, chest, shoulders, and face.

The breath of fire should be practiced slowly at first. As your confidence grows, the speed should be
increased. In general, beginners who are uncertain can use the long deep breath instead of the breath
of fire. During menstruation and pregnancy the breath of fire should not be practiced and the long deep
breath should be used instead.

The breath of fire is an essential element of KUNDALINI YOGA. This rhythmic and continuous diaphragm breathing is utilized in many asanas. In a short amount of time, the body is enriched with prana. In this manner, body and soul are quickly cleansed and energized.

With regular practice, you can greatly increase your lung capacity in a short amount of time, which is very helpful for particular meditations and strenuous Yoga practices.

Circulation increases and the nervous system is strengthened. In this way, the body is instantly detoxified; toxins in the lungs, airways, blood vessels, and blood cells are eliminated. In the case of serious poisons in the body—for example, drugs, nicotine, or caffeine—your condition can worsen first, such as with spells of dizziness. In this event, the breath should be relaxed for a moment. This breath technique is frequently practiced for afflictions of the blood, such as circulatory problems. With a correct employment of the breath of fire, the oxygen levels in the blood remain about the same (which distinguishes it from hyperventilation).

LEFT AND RIGHT NOSTRIL BREATHING
NADHI SODHANA

Sit in the simple seated pose with your back straight. With your right thumb, close your right nostril and breathe long and deep through your left nostril into your stomach, chest, and up to the collarbones. Exhale in reverse order. Completely use your entire breath. After three minutes, close the left nostril with your index finger and breathe long and deep for another three minutes through the right nostril. Then repeat this breath cycle. During the entire exercise, concentrate on your third eye, and in your mind, let the mantra SAT resonate with each inhale and the mantra NAM resonate with each exhale.

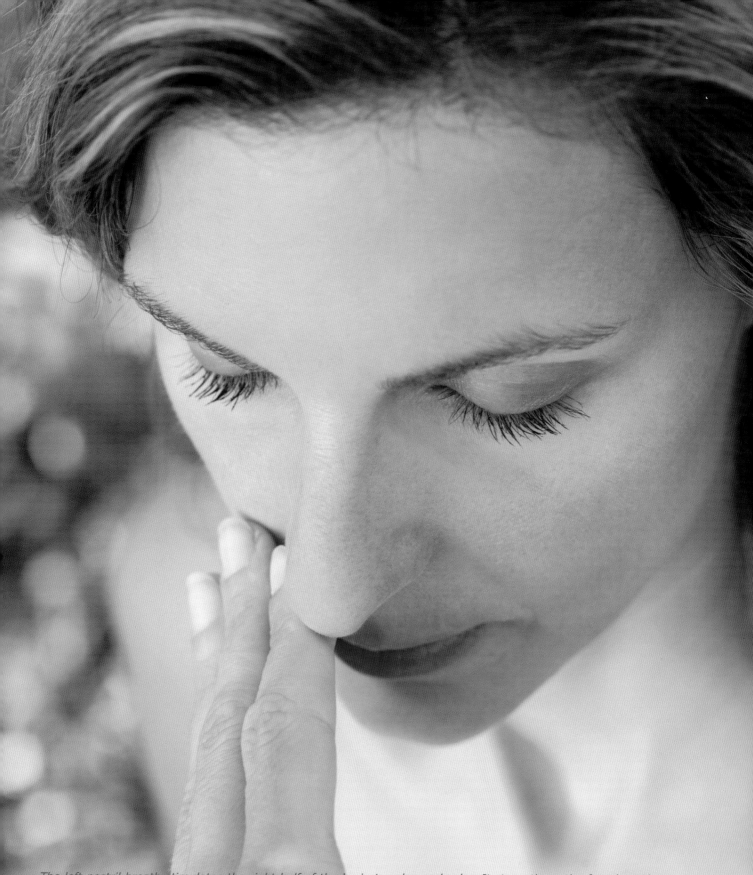

The left nostril breath stimulates the right half of the brain to relax and calm. It strengthens the female and the receptive, and promotes wisdom and intuition. It activates ida, the moon energy channel, and stimulates apana.

The right nostril breath has a stimulating and energizing effect. It promotes drive and will. The stimulation of the left half of the brain activates the male, the active, and the linear. It stimulates pingala, the sun energy channel, and mobilizes prana.

The intentional alternating of the breath cleanses body and mind and creates stability and clarity. It brings prana and apana into a harmonious balance.

COOLING BREATH
SITALI PRANAYAMA

Take a relaxed, seated position. Roll the tongue into a U shape and push it forward between the lips. If you cannot roll your tongue, push the tip of your tongue slightly between your lips. Breathe through the tongue deeply with a hissing, whistling noise. Concentrate on the cooling effect of the inhaled breath in your mouth and throat. Hold your breath briefly, and then exhale through the nose. Feel how the cool spreads through your entire body.

Finally, breathe in, hold your breath, pull in your tongue, and close your mouth. Exhale through the nose and relax. Perform this breath exercise twice for five minutes each time.

Sitali pranayama calms and cools the spine, in particular the area between the fourth and sixth vertebrae, where sexual and digestive energy get blocked. This exercise can also be used to lower a fever and to calm the brain and nervous system. With regular practice, it is very effective for detoxification and anti-aging. At first, a bitter taste may occur on the tongue. This is a sign that the detoxification process is occurring. With regular practice of this exercise, a sweet taste will eventually appear.

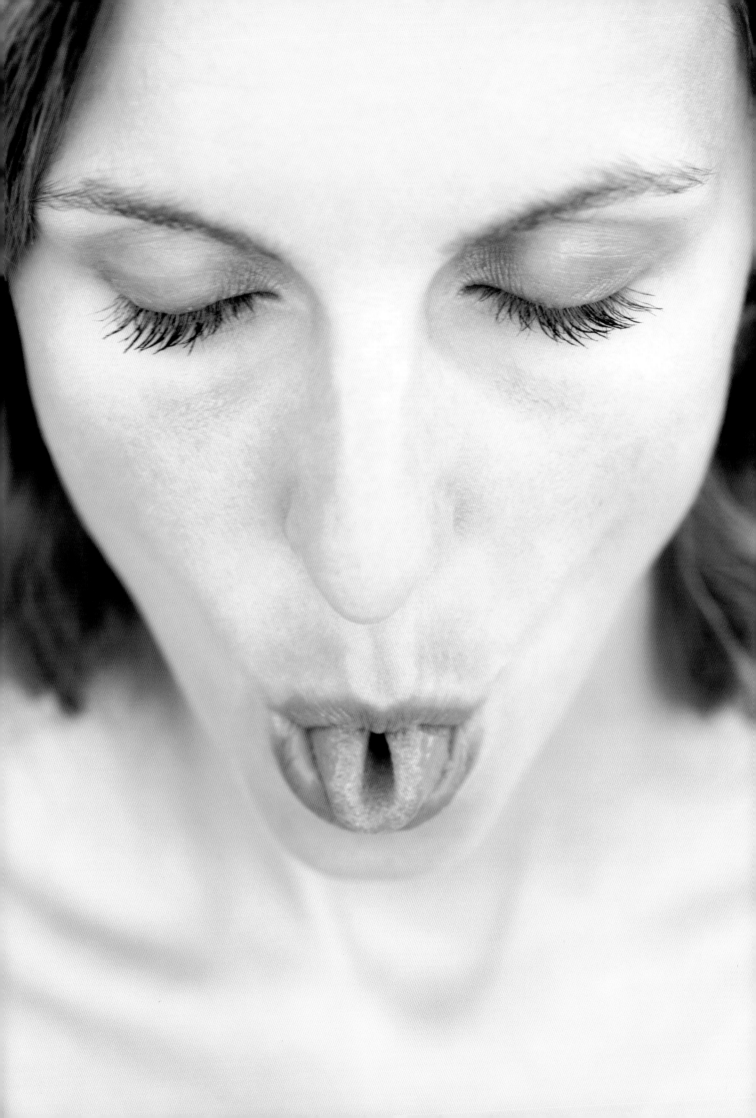

"Knowing only becomes true wisdom when you experience it with your own heart and being. Only the actual experience of this wisdom—gyan—can carry and support you." —Y. B.

# MUDRAS
MUD = JOY, GESTURE
RA = THAT, WHAT IS, WHAT PROJECTS

Mudras are "seals," symbolic hand gestures or movements that are used in many meditations and asanas. The various mudras create important energetic connections in the nervous system and stimulate particular nadis.

Every part of the hand is linked to a specific part of the brain. Bending, crossing, expanding, and touching the fingers or particular portions of the hand stimulates reflex zones and meridians, which has a direct effect on the body and mind. Particular symbols and elements are attributed to each finger. For example, the thumb stands for the ego and the element fire; pressure on the tip of the thumb stimulates the lung meridian.

Mudras have a meaningful influence on the mind of the person practicing. They deepen spiritual development and support the awakening of the Kundalini. The employment of mudras in meditative and dynamic asanas, as well as in meditation, strengthens their energetic effects.

GHYAN MUDRA
GHYAN = KNOWLEDGE, PERCEPTION

In the ghyan mudra, the tip of the thumb touches the tip of the index finger.

Symbol   Ego (thumb) and Jupiter (index finger)

Element   Fire (thumb) and air (index finger)

Meridian   Lung meridian (thumb) and large intestine meridian (index finger)

Effect   Grants awareness; stimulates intuition and receptiveness; promotes intelligence and mental growth

This mudra symbolizes the unification of the individual and universal souls and is the most utilized mudra in Yoga.

The planet Jupiter represents knowledge and its expansion, and it stands for the role of the protector. Any opposites are nobly harmonized; positive feelings can freely bloom. Jupiter energy grants confidence and strengthens inner harmony.

In many pranayamas and in specific exercises, the active variations of ghyan mudra are used. In this case, the index finger is bent so that the nail presses against the inner side of the upper thumb joint.

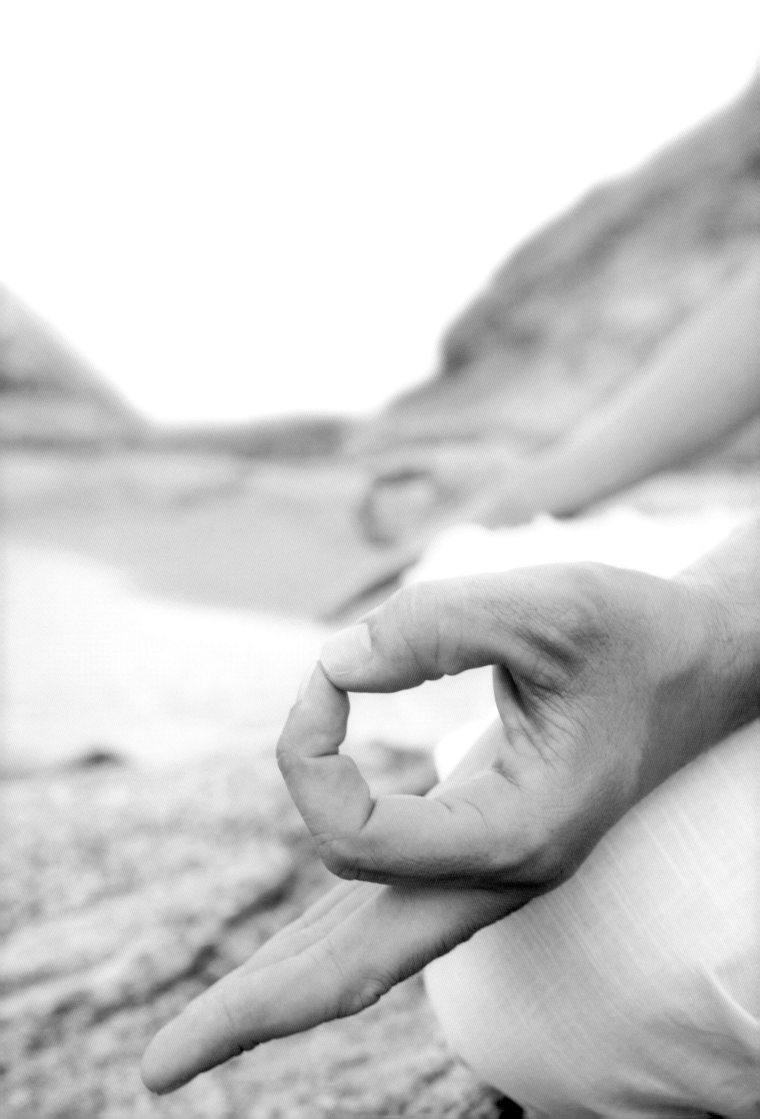

SHUNI MUDRA
SHUNI = PATIENCE

In the shuni mudra, the tip of the thumb touches the tip of the middle finger.

Symbol   Ego (thumb) and Saturn (middle finger)

Element   Fire (thumb) and sky (middle finger)

Meridian   Lung meridian (thumb) and pericardium meridian (middle finger)

Effect   Promotes discipline and patience; strengthens the relation to reality; strengthens judgment making and sense of responsibility

Saturn represents the overseer, the karmic law. It stands for responsibility and courage. It grants the ability to live, deepen, and learn from experience.

If Saturn's energy is harmoniously balanced, it allows analytical thought and restores a clear, goal-oriented mind.

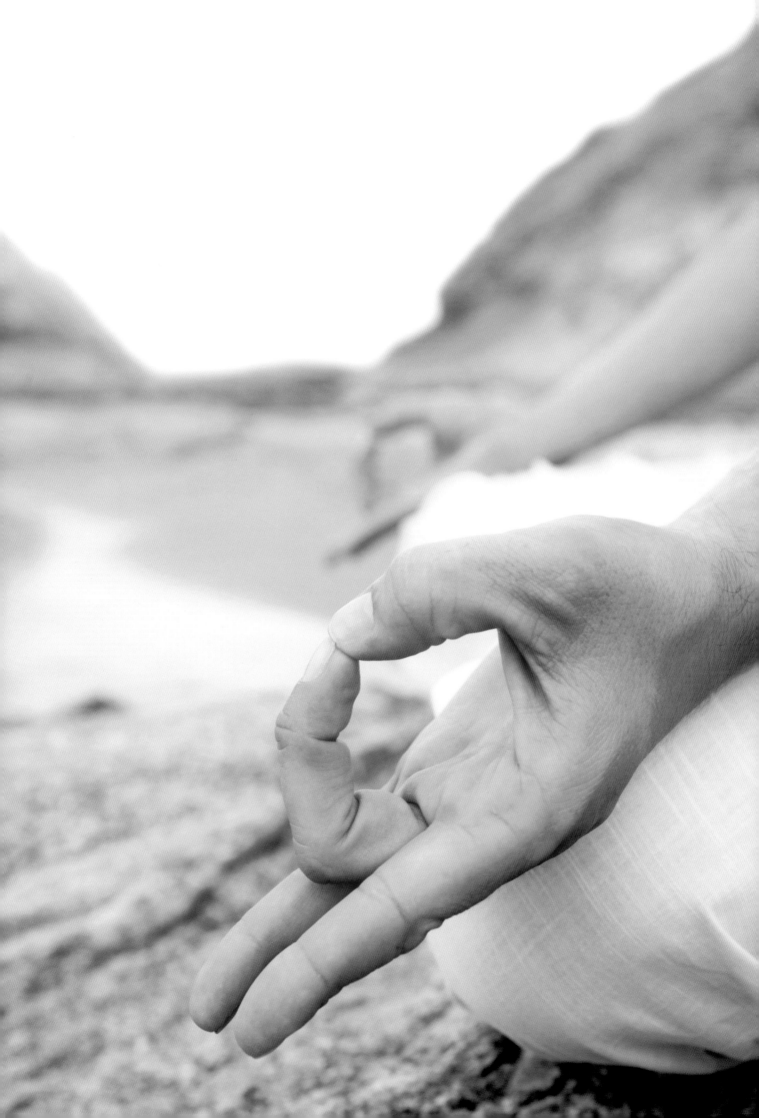

SURYA MUDRA
SURYA = SUN

In the surya mudra, the tip of the thumb touches the tip of the ring finger.

Symbol   Ego (thumb) and Sun/Uranus (ring finger)

Element   Fire (thumb) and earth (ring finger)

Meridian Lung meridian (thumb) and triple warmer meridian (ring finger)

Effect   Harmonizes energy and vitality; promotes health and strengthens the nervous system

The Sun represents energy, health, vitality, courage, will, nobility, and confidence. Uranus stands for the attainment of a higher consciousness. It influences the nervous system and intuition with its positive power. It promotes transformation, strengthens instinct, and energetically supports the mastery of all duties.

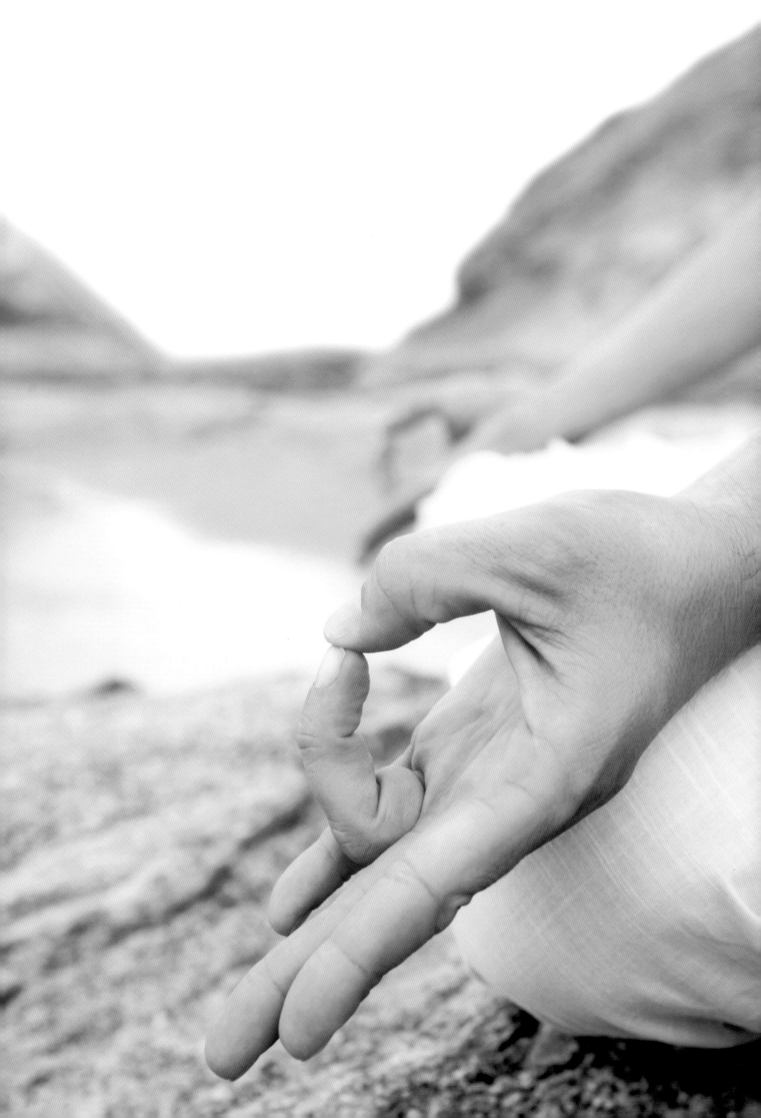

BUDDHI MUDRA
BUDDHI = COMMUNICATION

In the buddhi mudra, the tip of the thumb touches the tip of the little finger.

Symbol   Ego (thumb) and Mercury (little finger)

Element   Fire (thumb) and water (little finger)

Meridian   Lung meridian (thumb) and small intestine meridian (little finger)

Effect   Increases the ability to communicate clearly and intuitively

Mercury represents intelligence and memory. It promotes eloquence as well as the ability to communicate and reason.

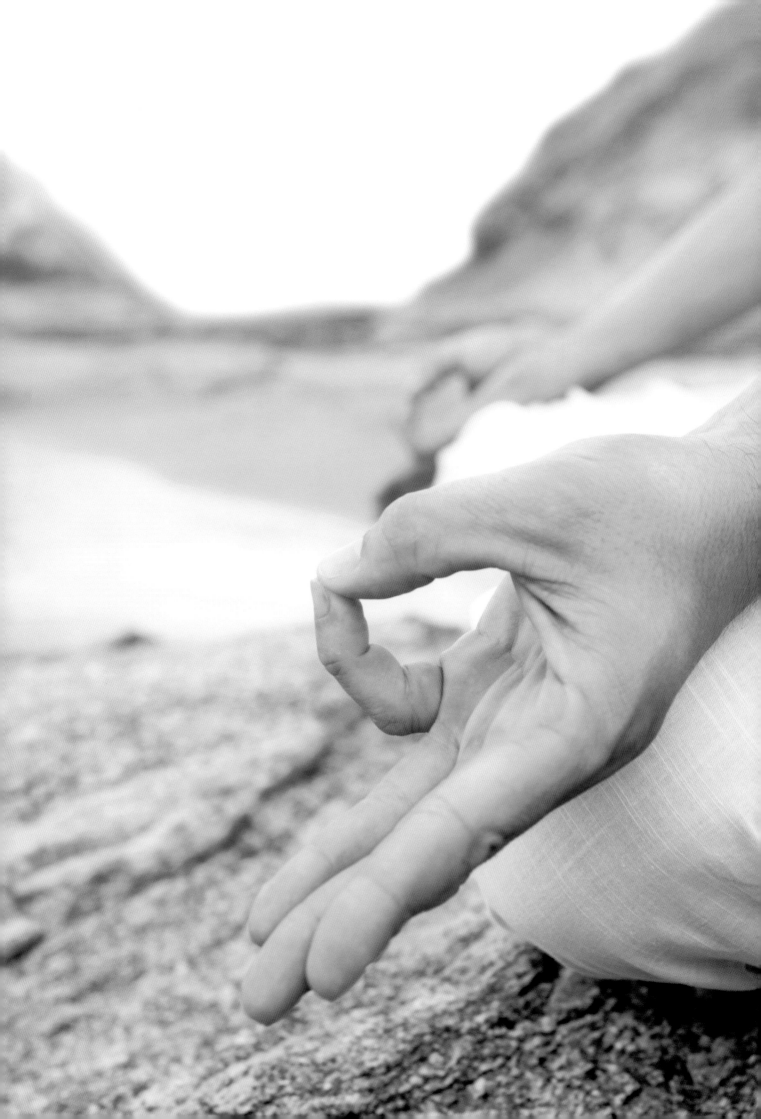

PRAYER POSE
PRANAM MUDRA

Place the hands together at chest height and lightly press the palms together. The thumbs exert gentle pressure on the sternum. Elongate the fingers and point them up and away from your body at an angle.

Through pressing the palms together, both halves of the brain are stimulated. A balance forms between the right, male side and the left, female side of the body. This is a vital condition for concentration.

The pressure of the thumbs on the sternum activates the heart chakra and the mind nerve, which runs directly from the heart to the brain and supports recollection. It helps to focus the thoughts and thus creates the basis for meditation.

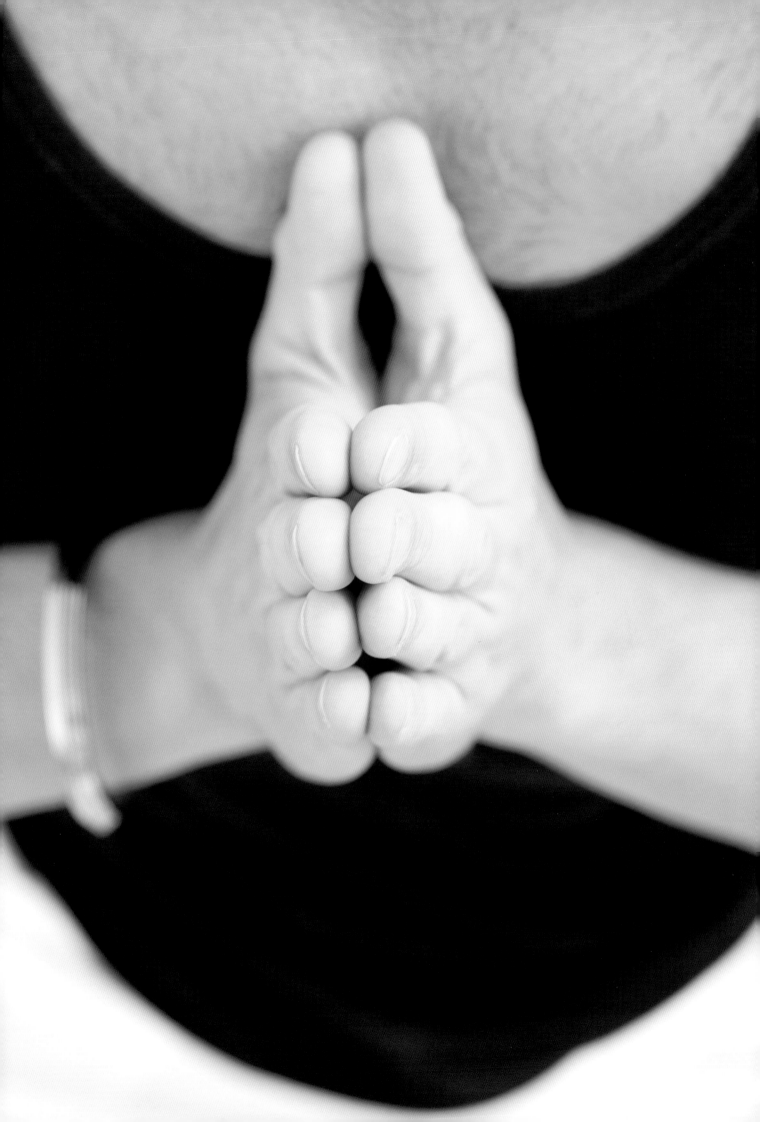

VENUS LOCK

Put your hands together and interlace your fingers.

Men should have the fingers of the right hand on top of the fingers of the left hand. The right thumb touches the Venus mound of the left hand (the mound above the base of the thumb). The left thumb lies in the space between the thumb and index finger of the right hand.

Women should have the fingers of the left hand on top of the fingers of the right hand. The left thumb touches the Venus mound of the right thumb. The right thumb lies in the spaces between the thumb and index finger of the left hand.

The name of this mudra comes from the way the thumbs touch the Venus mound of the opposite thumb. This mound symbolizes the planet Venus.

The Venus lock stimulates and harmonizes the energies in the sacral chakra and transforms them into higher levels. This grip refreshes, clarifies, aids concentration, and provides new motivating power.

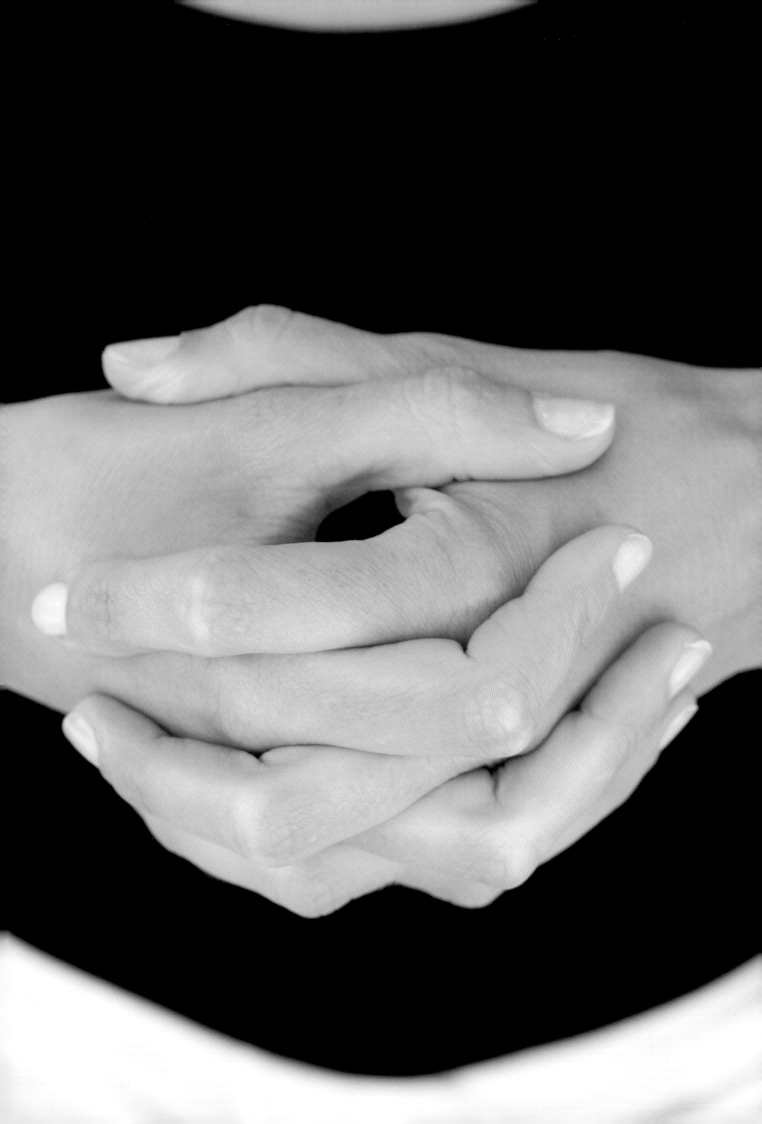

BEAR GRIP
GANESH MUDRA

Lift your arms horizontally to the sides and bend them so that both the forearms and upper arms are parallel to the floor. Bend the fingers and hook the hands together in front of the heart chakra. The right palm faces the chest, the left faces forward. Pull your arms apart strongly, without losing your grip. Make sure that the arms and shoulders remain relaxed.

This mudra opens and energizes the heart chakra. It stimulates the thymus gland, strengthens the immune system and the lymphatic system, and activates self-cleansing and concentration.

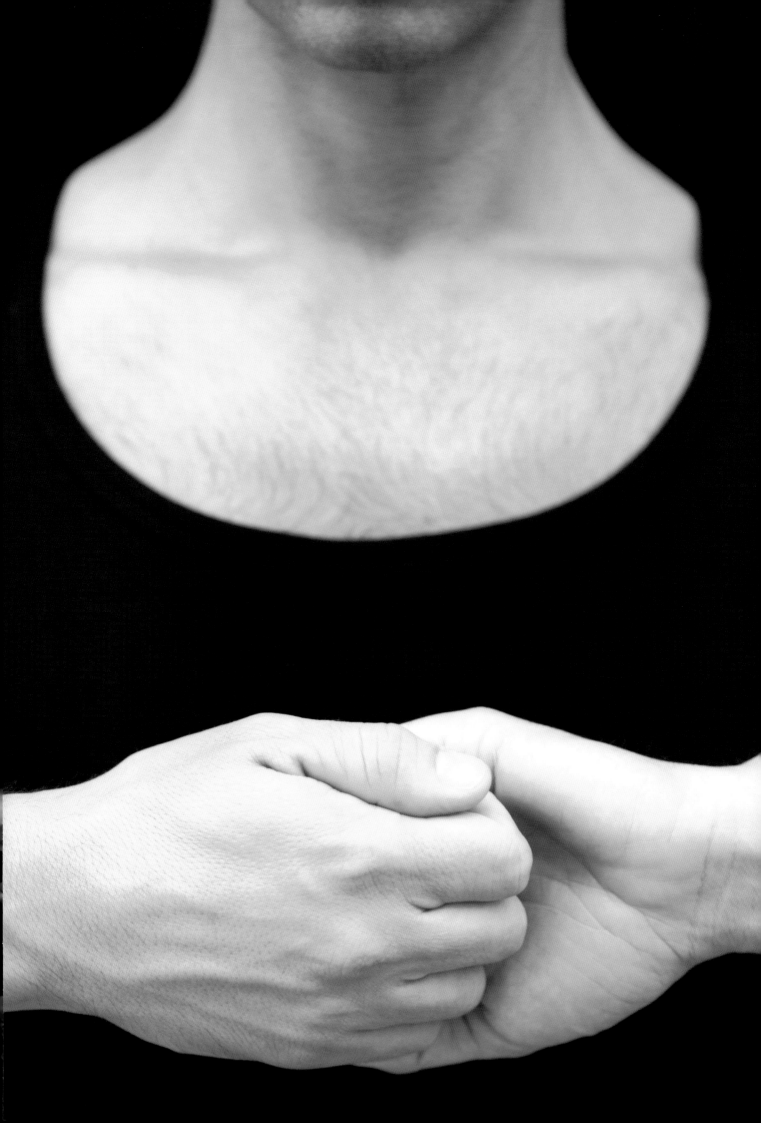

"The Universe has given us life and the best thing that we can do is to love life and to be happy. In Kundalini Yoga we unfurl our sleeping energy so we can lead a fulfilled, intuitive, and admirable life in a normal life situation, as a part of this world." —Y. B.

CHAKRA
CHAKRA = WHEEL, DISCUS, CIRCLE

Chakras are psychoenergetic hubs along the spinal column. When these energy fields are activated, they open and turn like wheels. When they are activated, they collect, transform, and distribute their inherent subtle and physical energies.

There are seven main chakras, each of which is assigned to physical functions and energetic qualities. The chakras are connected with each other via the sushmana, the main energy channel for the Kundalini. According to Yogi Bhajan, the aura comprises the eighth chakra and appears due to the combined effects of the seven main chakras.

To bring body and mind into a harmonious balance, it is necessary to open the chakras. Blocked energy hubs, when either closed or only slightly opened, can bring about physical and psychic dysfunction or insensitivities.

Asanas and meditation in KUNDALINI YOGA help to activate and open the chakras in many ways and thus to remove physical and energetic blocks.

1. CHAKRA: ROOT CHAKRA (MULADHARA)
MULA = ROOT, SOURCE, ESSENCE
ADHARA = BASE, FOUNDATION, SUPPORT

The root chakra is located at the lower end of the spinal column between the anus and genitals and is connected to the tailbone.

Color	Red (vitality)
Symbol	Four-petaled lotus
Element	Earth (prithivi): Mother, power, nourishment, security, protection
Planet	Mars
Plexus	Sacral Plexus
Prana	Apana (elimination)
Sensory Organ	Nose (smell)
Bodily Attribution	Pelvic floor, large intestine and colon, bones, legs and feet, teeth and nails, blood formation, digestion, sciatic nerve
Attributed Glands	Adrenal glands
Physical Function	Bone/tooth/nail growth, digestion, elimination
Physical Dysfunction	Intestinal disease, constipation, diarrhea, lower back pain, lumbago, sciatic pain, bone disease, osteoporosis, pain in the legs and feet, stress-induced illness, weak constitution
Psychic Function	Stability, vitality, will to live, primal instinct, ability to follow through, self-confidence, self-absorption, grounding
Psychic Dysfunction	Weakness, little joy for life, lack of trust in life, existential fear, suspiciousness, depression, lack of grounding

2. CHAKRA: SACRAL CHAKRA (SVADHISTHANA)
SVADHISTHANA = SWEETNESS, LOVELINESS

The sacral chakra is located above the genitals, on the border between the tailbone and sacrum.

Color	Orange (activity, energy, happiness, hope)
Symbol	Six-petaled lotus
Element	Water (apas): softness, flexibility
Planet	Mercury
Plexus	Sacral plexus
Prana	Apana (elimination)
Sensory Organ	Tongue (taste)
Bodily Attribution	Pelvic area, sacrum, sex and pelvic organs, uterus, kidneys, spleen, bladder, prostate, hip joints, lumbar spine
Attributed Glands	Gonads, adrenal glands
Physical Function	Activation of sexual and reproductive function, detoxification, circulation, lymphatic flow, immune system
Physical Dysfunction	Menstrual discomfort, sexually transmitted disease, kidney disease, bladder problems, urinary tract infections, lumbar pain, hip pain, effects of a lack of detoxification
Psychic Function	Sexuality, sensuality, reproduction, feelings, creativity, enthusiasm, eroticism, creative life energy
Psychic Dysfunction	Inability to enjoy life, psychic weakness, lack of motivation, jealousy, feelings of guilt, disturbed sexual behavior (addiction, disinterest), powerful mood swings

3. CHAKRA: NAVEL CHAKRA (MANIPURA)
MANIPURA = LUMINOUS JEWEL

The navel chakra is located about two fingers' widths beneath the belly button.

Color	Yellow (fire, energy)
Symbol	Ten-petaled lotus
Element	Fire (tejas): digestive fire, cleansing
Planet	Sun
Plexus	Solar plexus
Prana	Samana (distribution of nourishment)
Sensory Organ	Eyes (sight, visualization)
Bodily Attribution	Stomach, small intestine, liver, spleen, gallbladder
Attributed Glands	Pancreas
Physical Function	Digestion, vegetative nervous system
Physical Dysfunction	Stomach/liver/spleen/gallbladder illness, digestive issues, lumbar pain, nervous disorders, diabetes, obesity
Psychic Function	Willpower, power, growth of the positive ego, self-control, self-awareness, drive, authority, inner balance, intuition, liveliness, strong nerves
Psychic Dysfunction	Lack of self-awareness, melancholy, frigidity, disinterest, blocked feelings, insecurity, lack of concentration, obsession with power, lack of life energy, recklessness, fits of rage, eating disorders, sleep disorders, not reaching goals, little assertiveness

4. CHAKRA: HEART CHAKRA (ANAHATA)
ANAHATA = UNTARNISHED, UNSPOILED

The heart chakra is located in the center of the chest at the height of the heart.

Color	Green
Symbol	Twelve-petaled lotus
Element	Wind (vayu): movement, energy, touch, emotion
Planet	Venus
Plexus	Cardiac plexus
Prana	Prana (breath)
Sensory Organ	Skin and hands (touch)
Bodily Attribution	Heart, lungs, bronchia
Attributed Glands	Thymus gland
Physical Function	Heart and lung function, circulation, blood pressure
Physical Dysfunction	Heart illness, arrhythmia, difficulty breathing, lung illness, blood pressure fluctuation, higher cholesterol level, blood flow disturbances, thoracic and shoulder pain
Psychic Function	Unconditional love, empathy, affection, healing, taking responsibility, loving accepting of self
Psychic Dysfunction	Emotional frigidity, lovelessness, taciturnity, bitterness, relationship difficulties, loneliness

5. CHAKRA: THROAT CHAKRA (VISHUDDA)
VISHA = IMPURITY, POISON
SHUDHHA = CLEANSING

The throat chakra is located in the area of the throat.

Color	Light blue
Symbol	Sixteen-petaled lotus
Element	Ether (akasha): space
Planet	Jupiter
Plexus	Carotid plexus
Prana	Udana (supports solid and liquid ingestion)
Sensory Organ	Ears (hearing)
Bodily Attribution	Neck, throat, jaw, esophagus, trachea, cervical spine
Attributed Glands	Thyroid gland
Physical Function	Breath, voice, aerobic metabolism
Physical Dysfunction	Neck pain, inflammation of the throat, mouth, gums, and jaw, hoarseness, speech disorders, cervical spine pain, thyroid malfunction
Psychic Function	Verbal and creative self-expression, eloquence, communicative ability, conscious word choice, inspiration, openness
Psychic Dysfunction	Difficulty with emotional and verbal expression, fear of giving your own opinion, reclusiveness, restraint, shyness, no access to the inner voice, speech disorders

6. CHAKRA: BROW CHAKRA (AJNA)
AJNA = PERCEPTION

The brow chakra is located between the eyebrows.

Color	Dark blue
Symbol	Ninety-six-petaled lotus (48 petals times two)
Element	Mind (manas)
Plexus	Medulla Oblongata
Prana	Samana (distribution of nourishment)
Sensory Organ	Third Eye (wisdom, intuition)
Bodily Attribution	Eyes, ears, paranasal sinuses
Attributed Organs	Pituitary gland
Physical Function	Regulation of the hormone and nervous systems, ability to memorize and concentrate
Physical Dysfunction	Headache and migraine, eye complaints, ear complaints, chronic colds, inflammation of the sinuses, nervous system illness, neurological disturbances and illnesses
Psychic Function	Intuition, willpower, extrasensory perception (telepathy), imagination, fantasy, mental clarity, self-awareness
Psychic Dysfunction	Concentration and learning impairment, lack of insight, lack of fantasy, no vision for the spiritual, unsettled mind

7. CHAKRA: CROWN CHAKRA (SAHASRARA)
SAHASRARA = THE THOUSANDFOLD

The crown chakra is located on the crown of the head, the highest point of the head.

Color	Violet
Symbol	Thousand-petaled lotus
Element	Soul (Brahma-loka)
Plexus	Cerebrum (brain)
Bodily Attribution	Midbrain
Attributed Glands	Pineal gland (epiphysis)
Physical Function	No correlation to specific organs, but rather a protective and supportive function for the entire organism
Physical Dysfunction	Immune impairment, nervous affectation, paralysis, sleep disorders
Psychic Function	The seat of the soul, spiritual understanding, universal awareness, self-actualization, inner peace, enlightenment (assuming that all other chakras are also fully developed and free of blockages)
Psychic Dysfunction	Entrapment in the material world, discontent, aimlessness, weltschmerz, feeling of emptiness, mental exhaustion, fear of death, denial of creativity

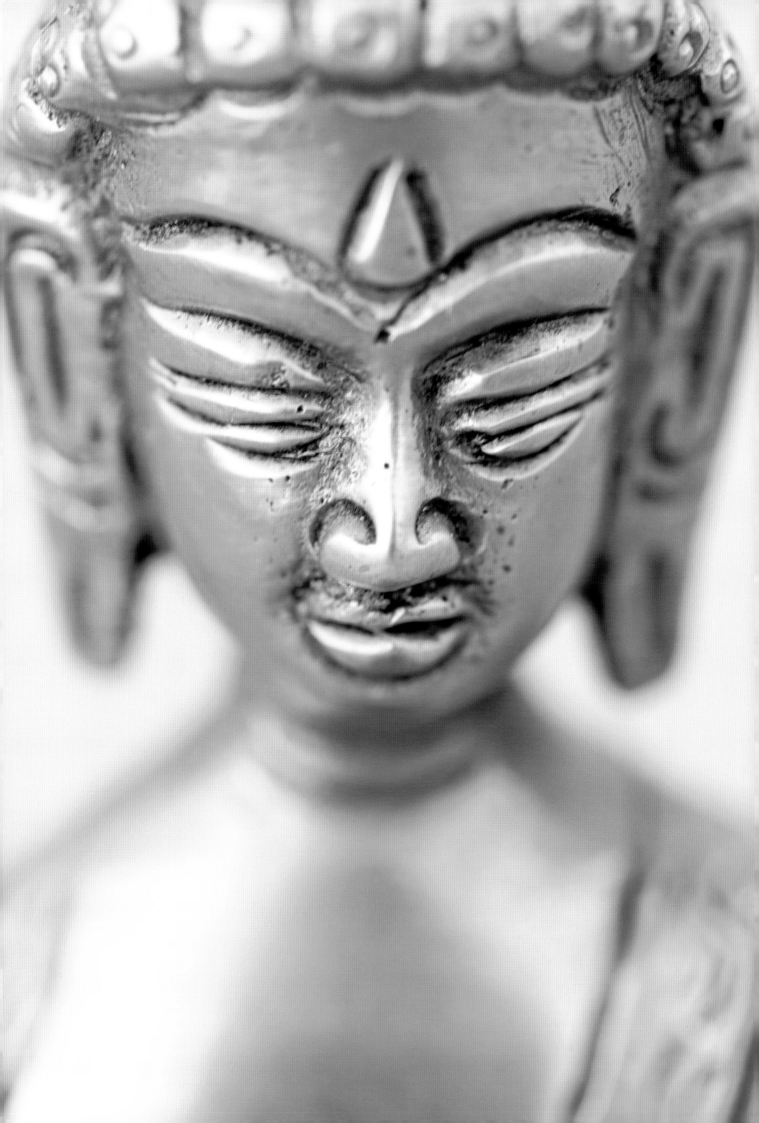

"We do not do Kundalini Yoga to become saints; we do it to experience our humanity." —Y. B.

BANDHA
BANDHA = LOCK

Bandhas are body locks at the key points on the body at which prana and apana flow together. These can be used by contracting specific muscle groups. The so-called engaging of the bandhas directs prana into the nadis. This stimulates the nervous system as well as the flow of spinal fluid and optimizes circulation and energy balance.

Engaging the bandhas is a fundamental aspect of Yoga and should be done as often as the exercises allow.

ROOT LOCK (MULA BANDHA)
MULA = ROOT, BASE, ORIGIN

As the most complicated of the three locks, mula bandha is a kind of hydraulic lock at the bottom end of the spinal column. By engaging the root lock, you stimulate and bring balance to the energies in the anal area, the sex organs, and the navel point. Sexual energies are transformed into creative processes.

The main function of mula bandha is the connection of prana and apana in the navel point, as well as the channeling of the energies from the lower three chakras into the upper chakras.

Engage mula bandha by first contracting the muscles of the anus. Then tense the muscles of the sex organs and pull them upward. Finally, pull the navel point and lower abdominal wall toward the spine and upward, so that the anus and sex organs are pulled upward. Make sure that in this series and in all three groups, you engage mula bandha very firmly.

The root lock is implemented while holding the exhale, unless otherwise specified. Those who are pregnant or who have injuries in the pelvic or tailbone area should avoid engaging mula bandha.

DIAPHRAGM LOCK (UDDHYANA BANDHA)
UDDHYANA = RISE, SOAR

Engaging uddhyana bandha allows prana to flow up freely through sushmana. Engaging the diaphragm lock will activate the healing of many abdominal and stomach illnesses, because the stomach and intestines are massaged and stimulated by the movement. The diaphragm, along with the breathing and heart muscles, is strengthened.

Engage uddhyana bandha by first completely exhaling in a very upright position. Then pull the diaphragm up and the abdominal muscles toward the spine. To release the diaphragm lock, first relax the stomach and then inhale.

Uddhyana banda should not be practiced in the event of pregnancy, high blood pressure, or injuries or inflammation of the internal organs.

THROAT LOCK (JALANDHARA BANDHA)

JAL = WATER
JALAN = BRAIN SECRETIONS
DHARA = OPENING IN SEVENTH CHAKRA

Jalandhara bandha is the most used body lock in KUNDALINI YOGA. Engaging this lock allows a free flow of prana to the brain. It stimulates the thyroid, parathyroid, and pituitary gland and regulates their functions.

To engage jalandhara bandha, stretch the neck vertically and pull it back while sitting in an upright position. Pull the chin in towards the throat, but make sure that your head does not tilt forward.

Unless otherwise specified, the throat lock should be utilized during all meditative poses. Engaging jalandhara bandha should be avoided in the event of pituitary dysfunction, high blood pressure, and acute throat inflammation.

GREAT LOCK (MAHA BANDHA)

MAHA = GREAT

The great lock is when all three locks are engaged. Maha bandha regulates the nervous system, blood pressure, circulation, and all ductless glands.

"In Yoga, the most important thing is the experience. Your experience goes directly into your heart. Words cannot replace experience because the consciousness does not absorb them. You expand your consciousness to attain a greater understanding of honor and truth. Then you can plan your life as you wish, unhindered. You will bring creativity and infiniteness into all aspects of your daily life." —Y. B.

ASANA
ASANA = POSE, SEAT

Originally, asana meant both the sitting mat and the lotus position as the basic position for meditation.

Today, the word 'asana' indicates particular body poses and exercises. In Yoga, there is a total of 84 different asanas, as well as countless variations on these basics. This system of body poses was developed to strengthen the musculature, keep the body flexible and healthy, and to prepare the body ultimately for long, motionless sitting in meditation.

Through regular practice of the asanas, control of the body will be perfected and the flow of thoughts will be calmed. In this way, practice harmonizes body and mind.

It is important when executing the asanas to enter and leave the pose consciously. The correct breath technique is also of particular importance to the success of the poses and exercises.

According to Patanjali, asana is the third level of Ashtanga Yoga.

CAT-COW

Cat-cow is wonderfully appropriate as a warm-up for the entire spine. It invigorates and lengthens the back and neck musculature in both directions and strengthens the nervous system.

STRETCH POSE

Lie on your back and stretch out your arms next to your body. Stretch the legs slightly with knees, heels, and big toes touching. Pull in your belly button and make sure that the lumbar spine touches the floor during the entire exercise. Now engage the throat lock, lift the head, and look toward the toes. Now also lift your legs and arms about six inches. If you have trouble with your lumbar spine, you can place your hands under your pelvis as support, with palms facing downward. Breathe either long and deep or the breath of fire. If you have less experience, you can also raise one leg at a time or bend the knees slightly. Make sure that the body is engaged during the entire exercise.

The stretch pose improves body tension, tightens the abdominal muscles, and supports digestion. It strengthens and harmonizes the navel point as a hub for willpower, vitality, and stamina. The exercise gives power and strengthens personal assertiveness.

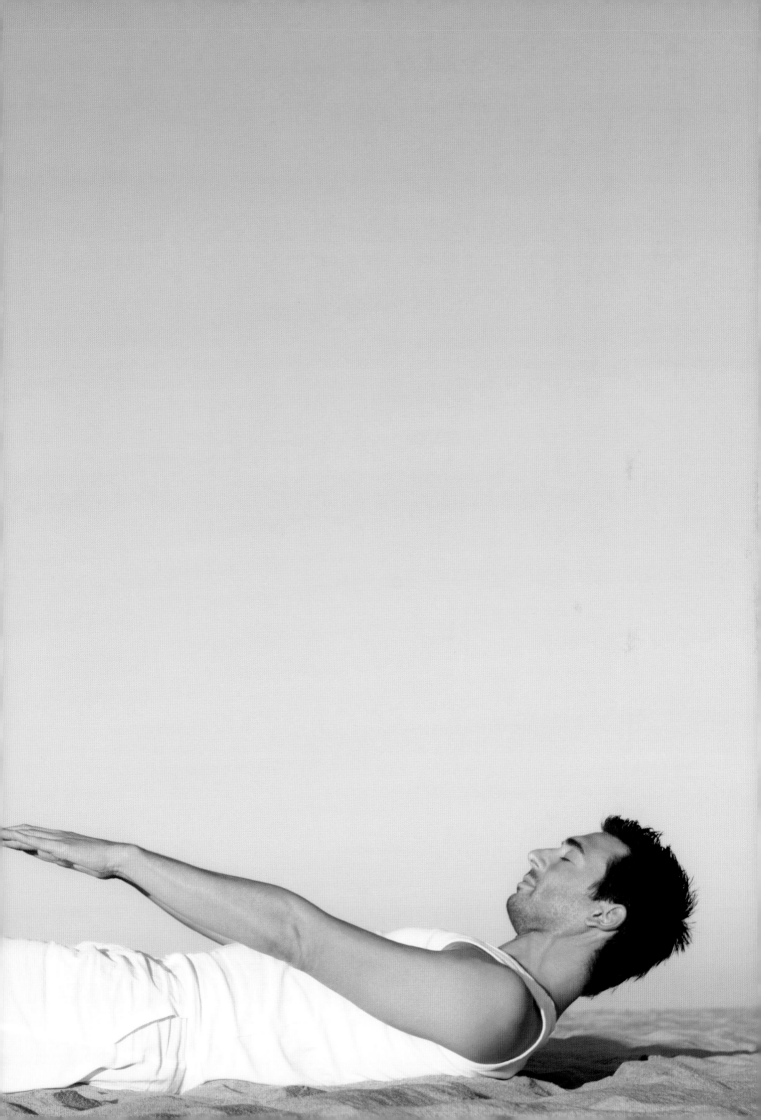

BABY POSE

The baby pose relaxes the spine and alleviates back pain. Circulation improves in the head and thyroid gland. The nervous system is calmed. The abdominal muscles are relaxed, the internal organs are massaged, and their function is regulated. The exercise removes fears and anxieties and grounds and strengthens the basic sense of trust.

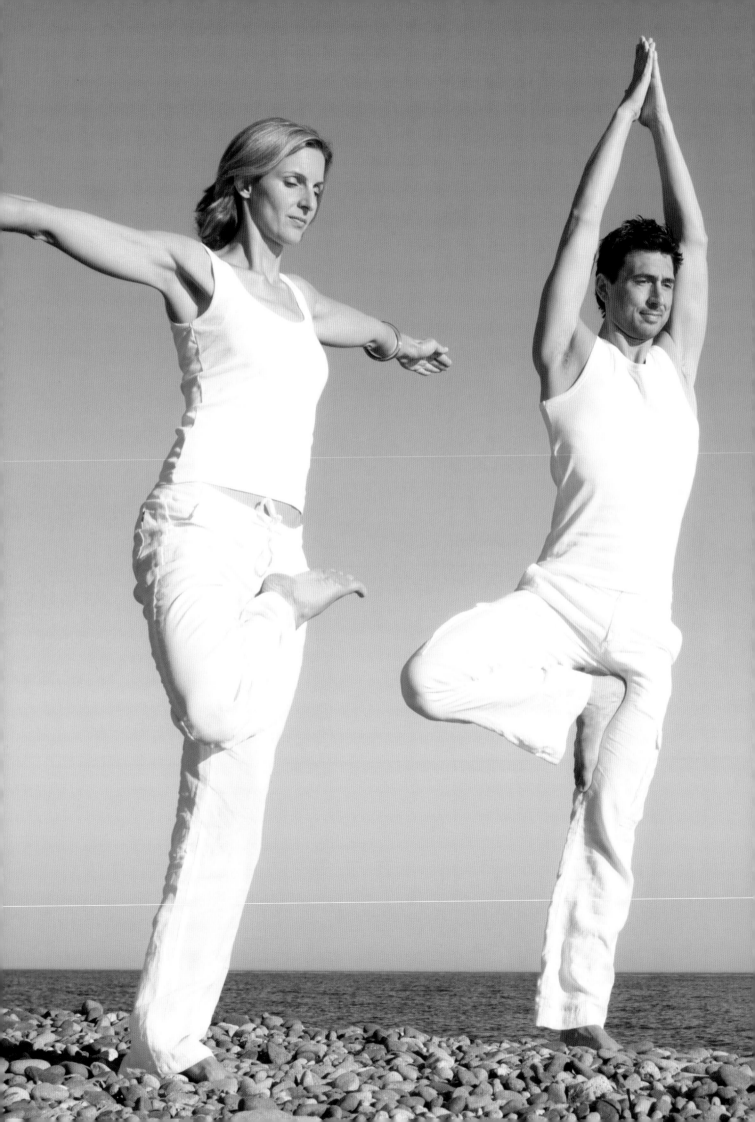

TREE POSE

Stand up straight, engage the throat lock, and shift your weight to your left foot. Lift the right leg and place your right foot on the inside of the left thigh near the groin, ideally as high as it can go. If you have less experience, you can also place your foot against the knee or calf. Now stretch your arms out horizontally to keep your balance. Look forward and fix your gaze on a specific point. When you feel securely balanced, you can stretch the arms up vertically. The upper arms touch the ears and the palms come together. Make sure that pelvis and shoulders face forward and are parallel and that the spine stays straight. During the entire exercise, engage mula bandha.

The tree pose steadies the leg and foot musculature and activates circulation in those areas. It relaxes the shoulders, expands the chest, and strengthens the pelvis and hips. In this way, the sense of balance and ability to concentrate are developed and supported.

KUNDALINI LOTUS

Sit upright with the throat lock engaged slightly and bring the soles of the feet together. Grasp your big toes with your index and middle fingers. In this position, lean back slowly until you can lift your feet from the ground. Your weight rests on the sitz bones. Slowly stretch out your legs to both sides until they form a 60° angle to the floor. To regulate balance, the belly button is drawn in. Make sure that your spine remains straight from tailbone to skull during the entire exercise.

The Kundalini lotus develops and strengthens the sense of balance. It aligns the pelvis, supports circulation through the sex organs, stretches the muscles in the backs of the legs and lower back, and invigorates the entire abdominal area.

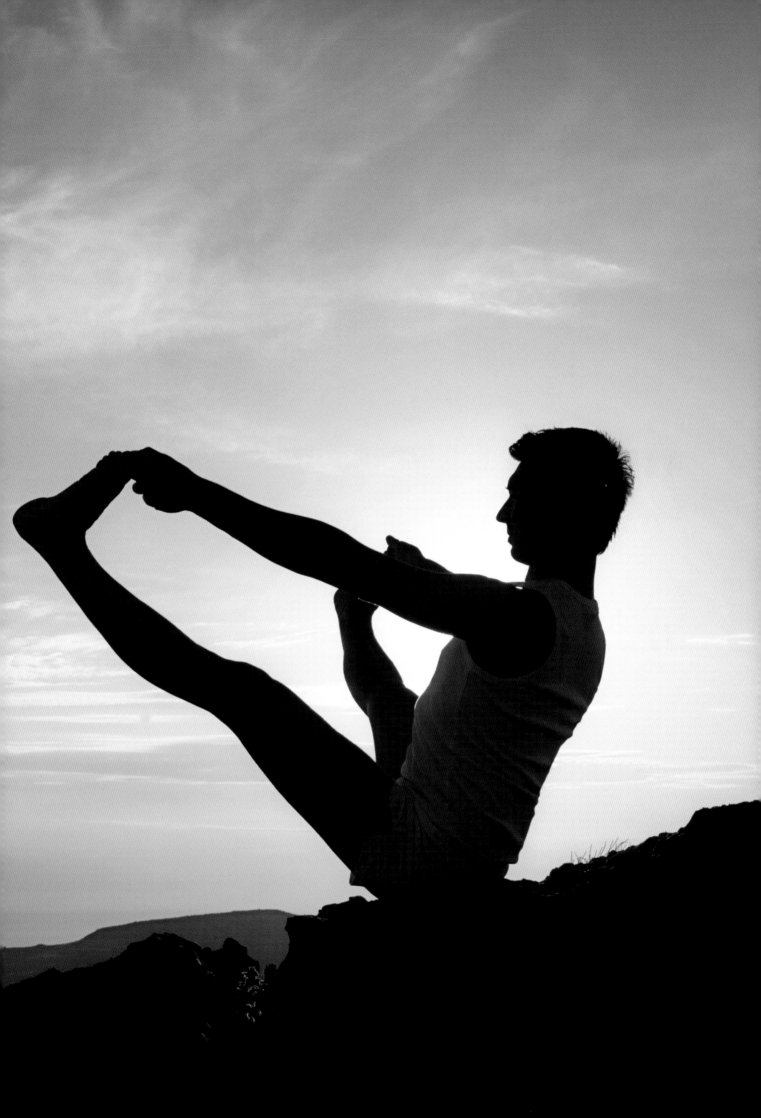

SPINAL TWIST

Sit in the simple seated pose with a straight back and engaged throat lock. Place your hands on your relaxed shoulders with the upper arms parallel to the floor and the elbows at shoulder height. Grasp the shoulders with the thumbs from behind and with the rest of the extended fingers from the front. From this starting position, turn the head and upper body to the left on the inhale, and to the right on the exhale. Make sure that the movement comes from the navel point and that the head does not turn farther than the body.

The spinal twist mobilizes and invigorates the spine. It strengthens the oblique abdominal muscles and the entire back musculature. At the same time, the abdominal cavity and lower body experience a gentle massage. This exercise helps sciatic, neck, and back discomfort and opens space for the chest, heart, and lungs. The heart chakra is activated, supporting compassion, love, and tolerance.

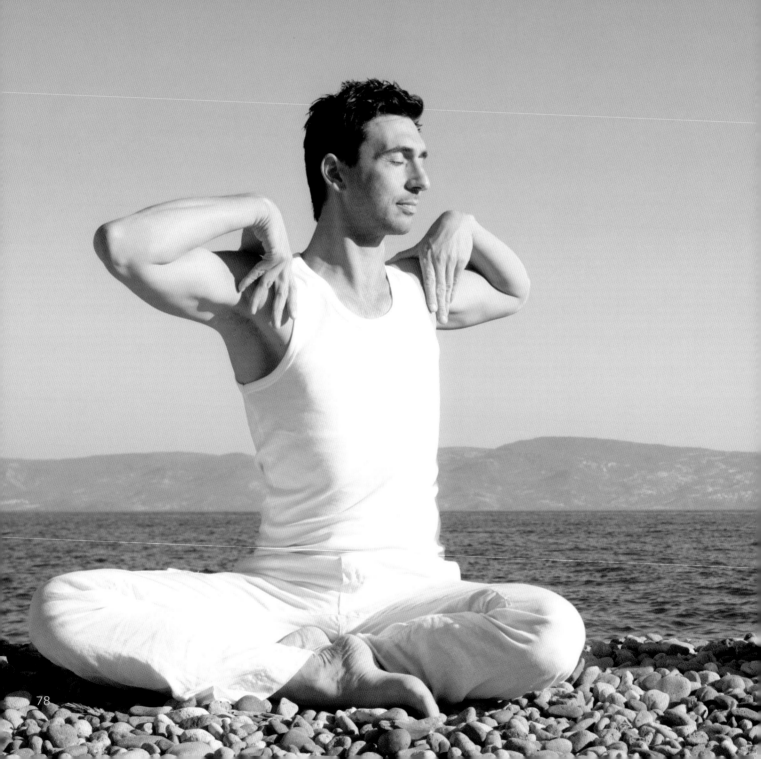

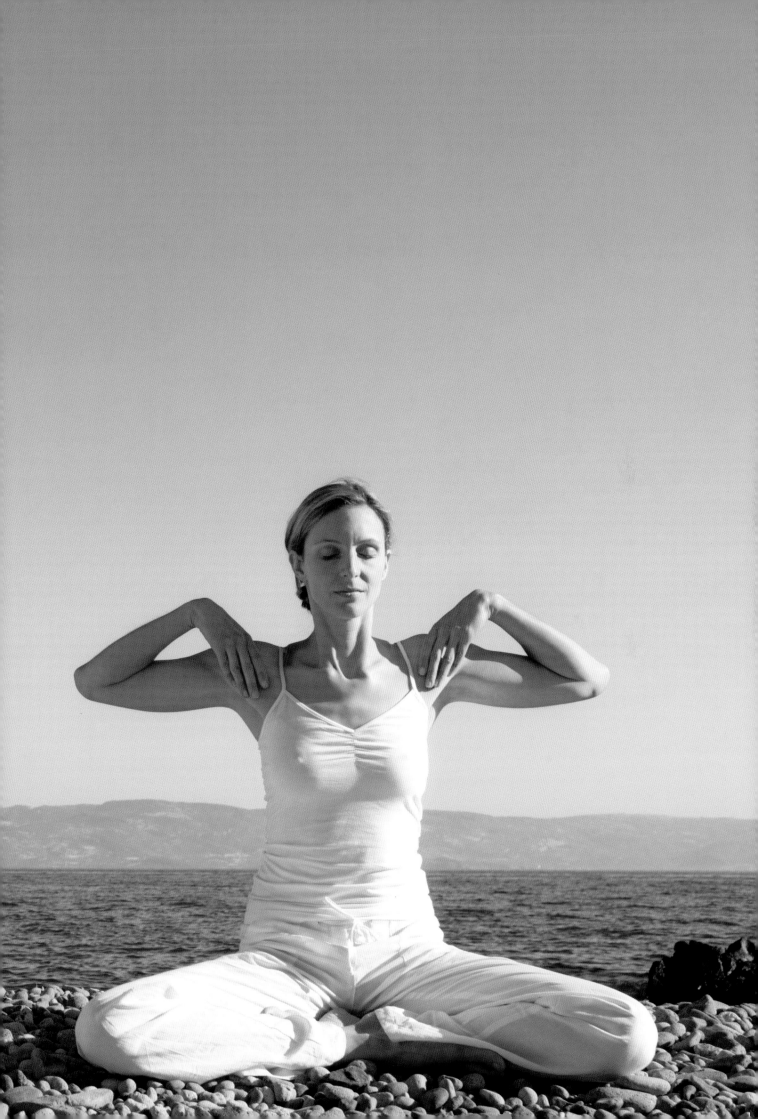

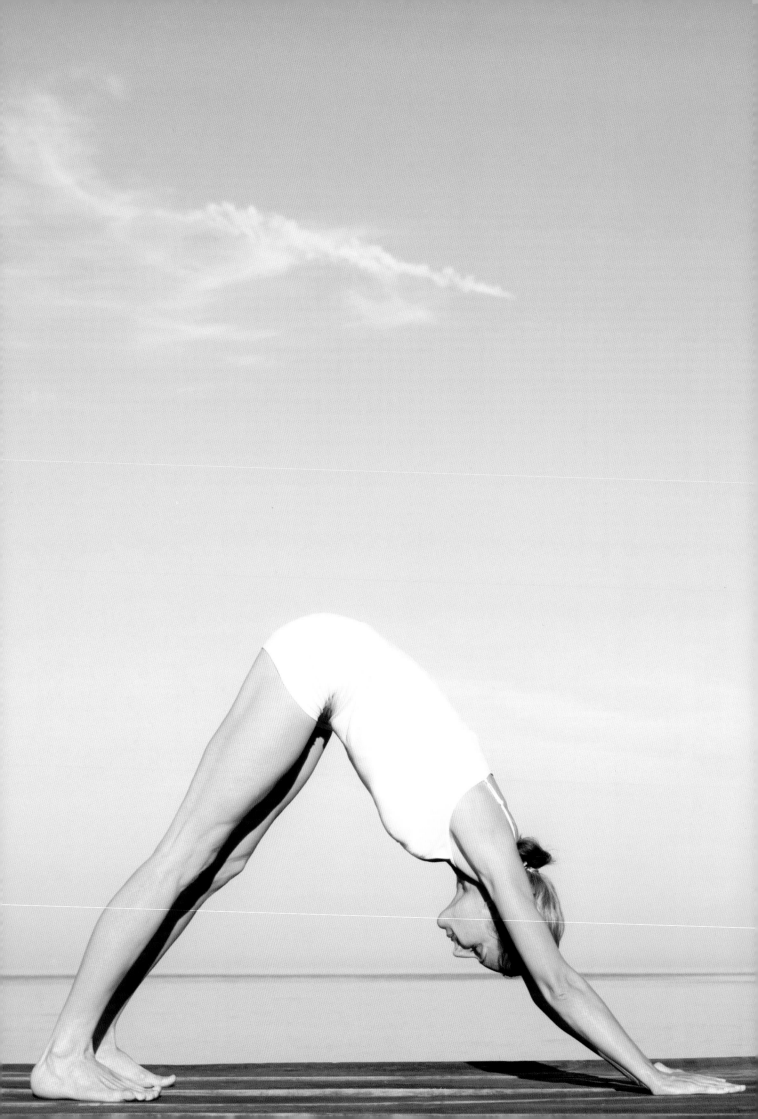

DOWNWARD DOG
TRIANGLE POSE

Lie on your stomach and place your hands under your shoulders. The fingers are spread and point forward with the thumbs pointing to each other. Make sure your elbows are next to your body. Set your feet hips' width apart, stretch out the arms, and lift your body off the floor. Lift the pelvis and extend the legs. Make sure that the sitz bones are the highest point of your body and that the spine creates a line with the extended arms. Relax the extended legs and set the heels on the floor. Distribute your weight evenly between hands and feet. Relax the head and neck area so that the chin leans slightly toward the chest. If you are experienced, you can come directly from the prone position to the downward dog.

The downward dog strengthens the entire back and arm musculature. It stretches the back, shoulders, and legs intensively. This exercise helps with osteoporosis, stiffness, and pain in the feet. It gives the entire body new energy. It has a calming effect on the heart and brain, lifts the mood during mild depression, relaxes in stressful situations, and strengthens the aura.

FORWARD BEND

Stand up straight with the legs together and stretch the arms up vertically on the inhale. On the exhale, pull the navel in and up, bend forward with a straight back, and lay the hands next to the feet on the floor. Alternatively, you can touch the floor with just the fingertips or you can grasp the calves. Keep the knees extended; bend them only if you have back problems. Make sure that the hips are directly above the heels and that your body weight is evenly distributed to both feet. Stretch the sitz bones and tailbone up and relax the neck and shoulders. Stretch the spine with each inhale and let gravity pull it lower on each exhale.

End the pose by slowly and carefully, vertebra by vertebra, returning the spine to the original position.

In the forward pose, the entire spine is simultaneously softly and intensively stretched. The internal organs are strengthened and massaged and digestive and menstrual discomfort is alleviated.

This exercise has a calming effect in stressful situations and helps with anxiety and sleeplessness.

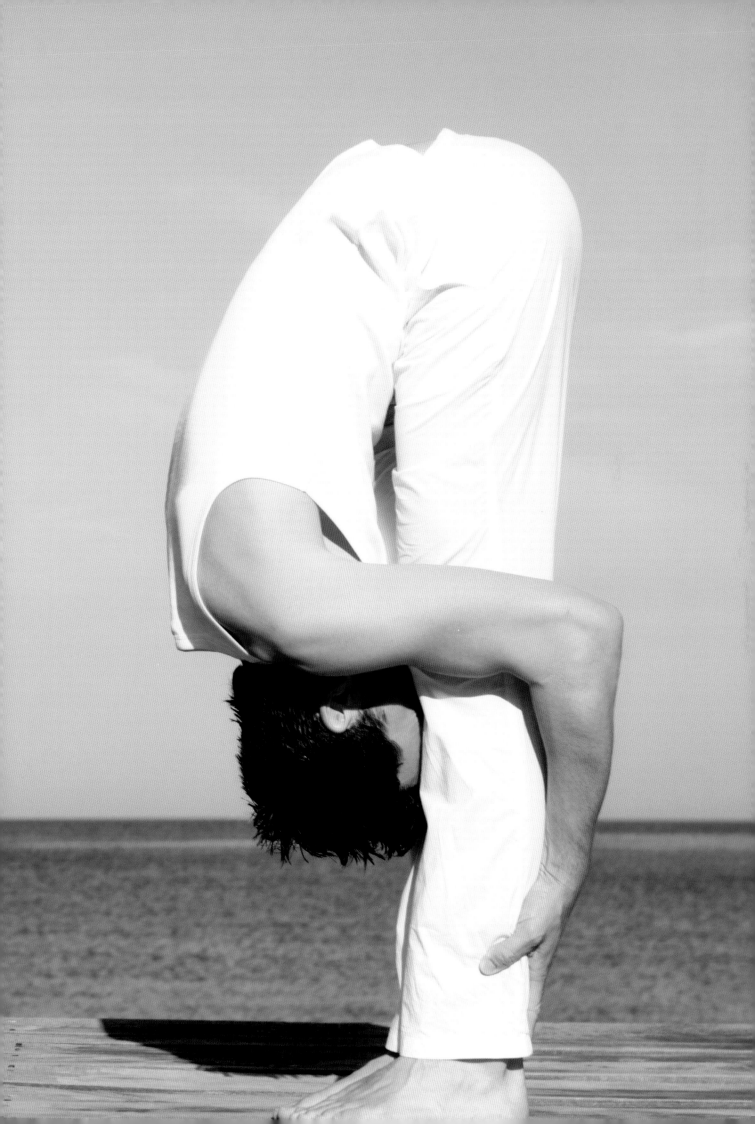

COBRA POSE

Lie on your stomach with your legs together and place your hands under your shoulders with palms facing the ground. Direct your gaze forward and lift your upper body by slowly stretching your arms. Only take this exercise as far as is comfortable for you. If you have experience, you can gently lay your head back on your neck and stretch your arms farther. Make sure not to raise the shoulders. The hip bones, legs, and tops of the feet touch the floor the entire time.

If you have problems with your lower back, you can substitute the simpler sphinx pose: lift the upper body from a prone position and support yourself on your forearms. The upper arms create a right angle with the floor and the palms face downward.

The cobra pose massages and strengthens the entire spinal musculature. It stretches the chest and lungs, activates the thyroid gland, strengthens the nervous system, and regulates digestion through pressure on the navel point. This exercise supports self-confidence. The heart center opens, and fears that are trapped inside are released.

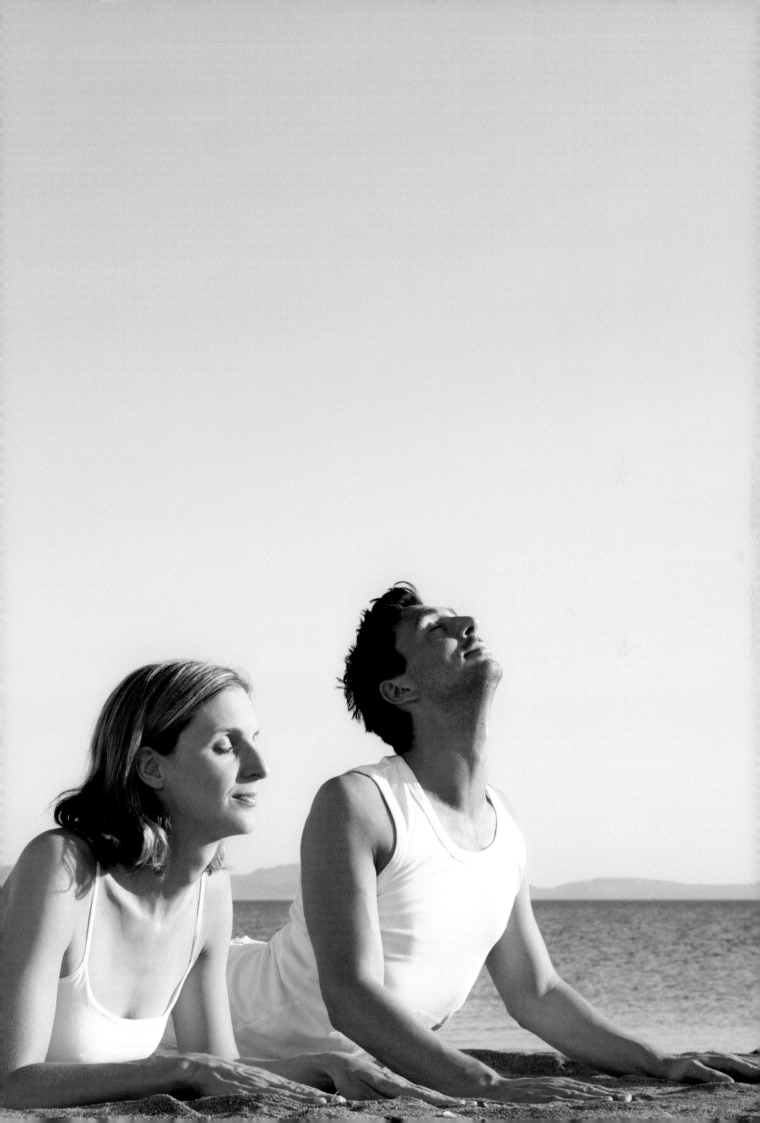

SHOULDER STAND

Lay on your back with your arms lying next to your body. Bend the knees and pull them to the chest while pressing the arms against the floor. Lift the pelvis and support it with the hands. The elbows remain shoulders' width apart during the entire exercise. Stretch the spine and legs straight up. Correct the pose by moving your hands toward the thoracic spine. Your weight rests on your shoulders and not on your neck. Make sure that you do not turn your head to the left or right.

End the pose by pulling the knees to the chest, removing your hands from your body and rolling slowly back into a supine position. Alternatively, you can move into plow pose.

The shoulder stand stimulates the thyroid gland, where the aerobic metabolism is regulated. As an inversion, this position has a simultaneously vitalizing and calming effect. It relaxes the brain and neck and normalizes digestion. It regulates the flow of prana and the function of the sex organs.

Shoulder stand should be avoided in the case of thyroid, neck, or menstruation problems, bad headache, high blood pressure, and during pregnancy.

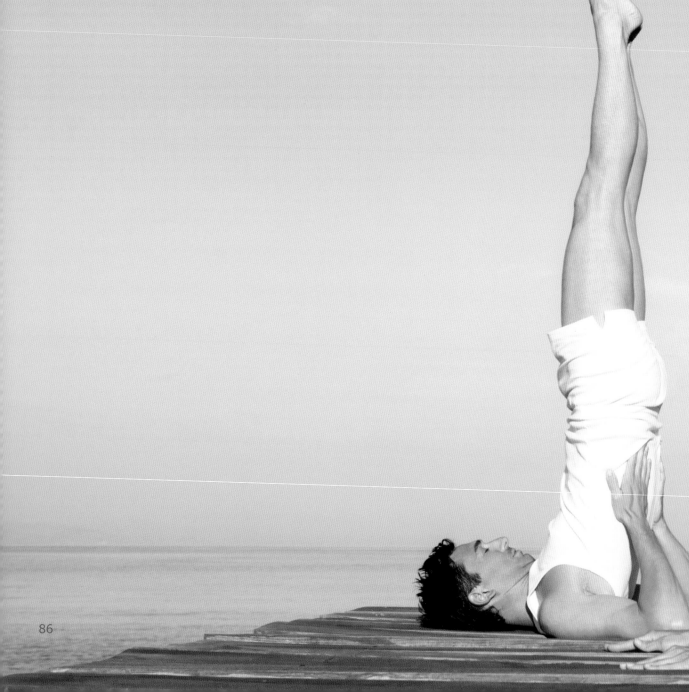

PLOW POSE

From the shoulder stand, lower the extended legs over the head and set the toes on the floor. While doing this, support your back with your hands. Pull the pelvis toward the feet and also up, so that your back becomes straight and stands vertically from the floor. Engage the throat lock. Stretch out the arms at shoulders' width with palms facing down, or interlace the hands in the Venus lock, and press them against the floor. If this is not possible for you, support your back instead. During this exercise, the knees are extended. If this is difficult for you, you can bend the knees and rest them on your forehead or next to your ears on the floor. Make sure that you do not turn the head to the left or right.

Finish the pose by bending the knees and rolling back, vertebra by vertebra, until you are lying stretched out on the floor again. Support your back so as to unburden the vertebral disks.

Like the shoulder stand, the plow is very effective for back discomfort. It stretches the entire spine and the shoulders, unburdens the internal organs, and regulates the function of the thyroid gland. This exercise activates circulation, helps with stress, headaches, and sleeplessness, and alleviates the symptoms of menopause.

The plow should be avoided in the case of herniated disks, heightened blood pressure, neck, thyroid, and heart problems, and during pregnancy or menstruation.

CAMEL POSE

Kneel up from the kneeling pose and place the knees hips' width apart. Engage the seat and abdominal musculature and bend back as far as possible. Make a circle backward with the right arm from the side of the body and support yourself with the hand on the right heel. Repeat the motion with the left arm and brace your left hand on your left knee. Stretch both the ribcage and the pelvis forward and pull the shoulder blades together. Make sure that the hips are directly above the knees. Relax your head back and concentrate on your third eye. During the entire exercise, engage mula bandha to avoid compression of the lumbar spine.

The camel pose achieves a high flexibility of the spine, ribcage, and lungs and strengthens the entire back, shoulder, and neck musculature. It massages the digestive organs and improves circulation in the kidneys and adrenal glands. In this way, it supports detoxification of the body.

The heart chakra opens and the ability to feel empathy is amplified.

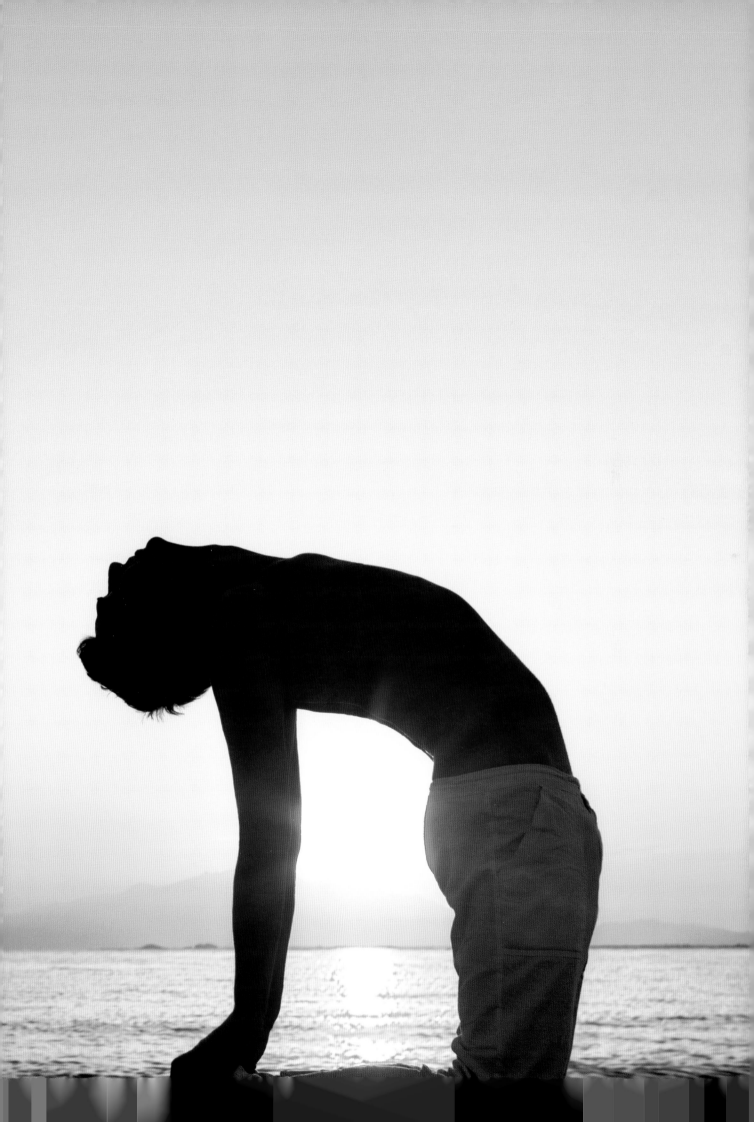

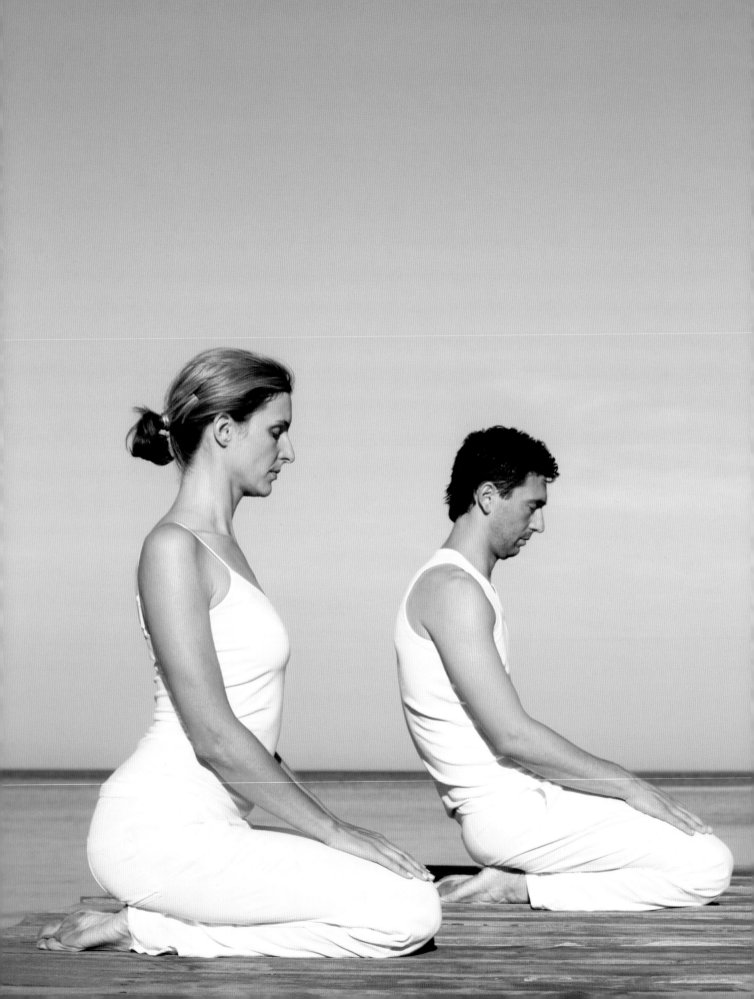

CAMEL RIDE
SPINAL FLEX

In the kneeling pose, lay the relaxed hands on the thighs. Inhale and arch your back as far forward and up as possible from the pelvis to the thoracic spine. Engage the throat lock. On the exhale, bend the entire spine back in the opposite direction. Repeat the movement. Make sure that the pelvis and head remain in the starting position and that only the back moves for the entire flow.

Camel ride promotes flexibility of the spine, strengthens and loosens the back and stomach musculature, and massages all of the internal organs. It improves physical and mental composure.

BOW POSE

Lie on your stomach and engage mula bandha. Bend the knees and grasp your feet or ankles behind your back. Engage the leg, seat, and lower back musculature and pull yourself up, so that your upper body and knees slowly leave the floor. Make sure that the knees remain hips' width apart. Hold mula bandha during the entire exercise to avoid compression of the lower back.

The bow pose mobilizes the entire spine. It strengthens the back musculature and protects against rheumatic discomfort. Through massaging the internal organs, the exercise stimulates appetite, promotes digestion, and helps with indigestion and gastro-intestinal problems. It stimulates the solar plexus, strengthens self-confidence, and elevates the mind.

This exercise should be performed carefully in the event of problems with the lower back or after abdominal surgery. The bow should not be practiced at all during pregnancy. The camel pose is recommended instead.

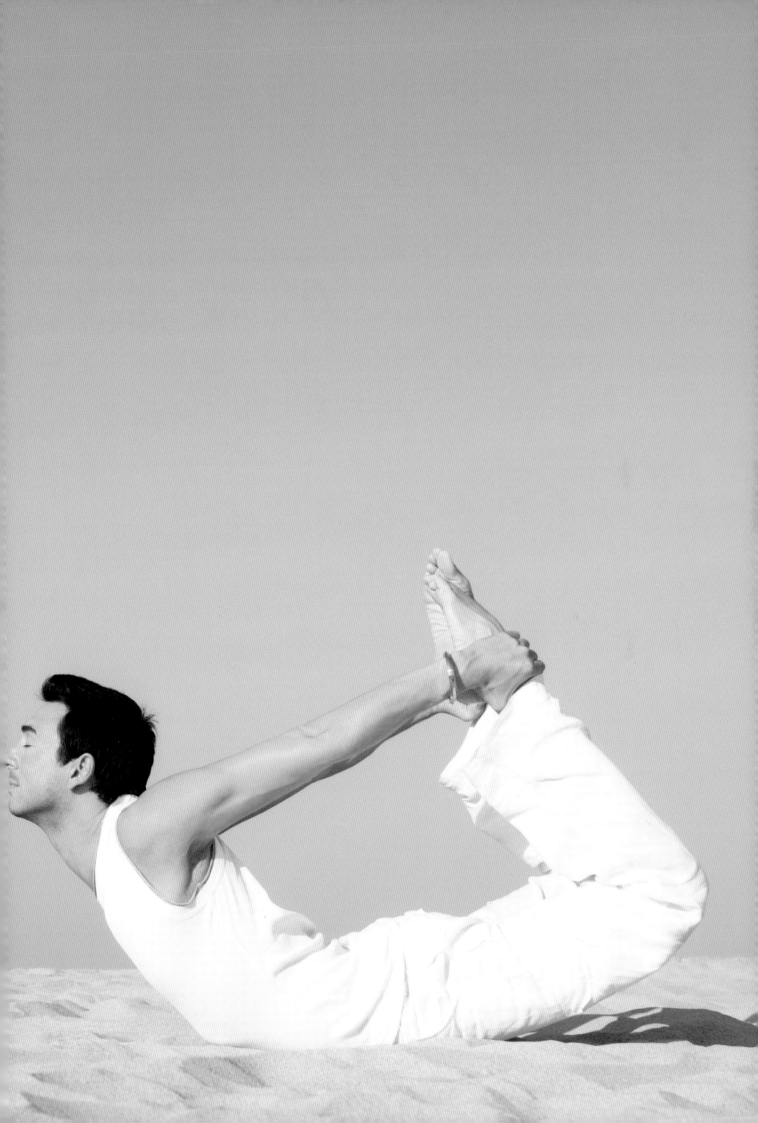

ARCHER POSE

While standing, step into a large lunge to the side with the right foot (25 to 40 inches according to body size). Turn the right foot 90° to the right so that it creates a line with the body. Turn the left foot 15° to the right. Shift your weight to the right foot and bend the leg until the knee is directly over the ankle. The left leg remains extended. The pelvis, hips, and upper body do not turn but rather remain in the original position for the entire exercise. Make sure to keep your upper body vertical and not to lean forward or backward.

Engage the throat lock. Relax the shoulders and stretch both arms out horizontally to the sides. Make fists with both hands; the thumbs point upward bend the left arm as if you were drawing a bow. Turn your head toward the right hand and fix your gaze on the crescent of your right thumbnail. Expand your chest by pulling both arms slightly back. Make sure that the arms remain parallel to the floor.

The archer pose strengthens the leg, back, and arm muscles, expands the chest and pelvis, and invigorates the nervous system.

It supports courage, self-confidence, and purposefulness and strengthens willpower, steadfastness, and assertiveness.

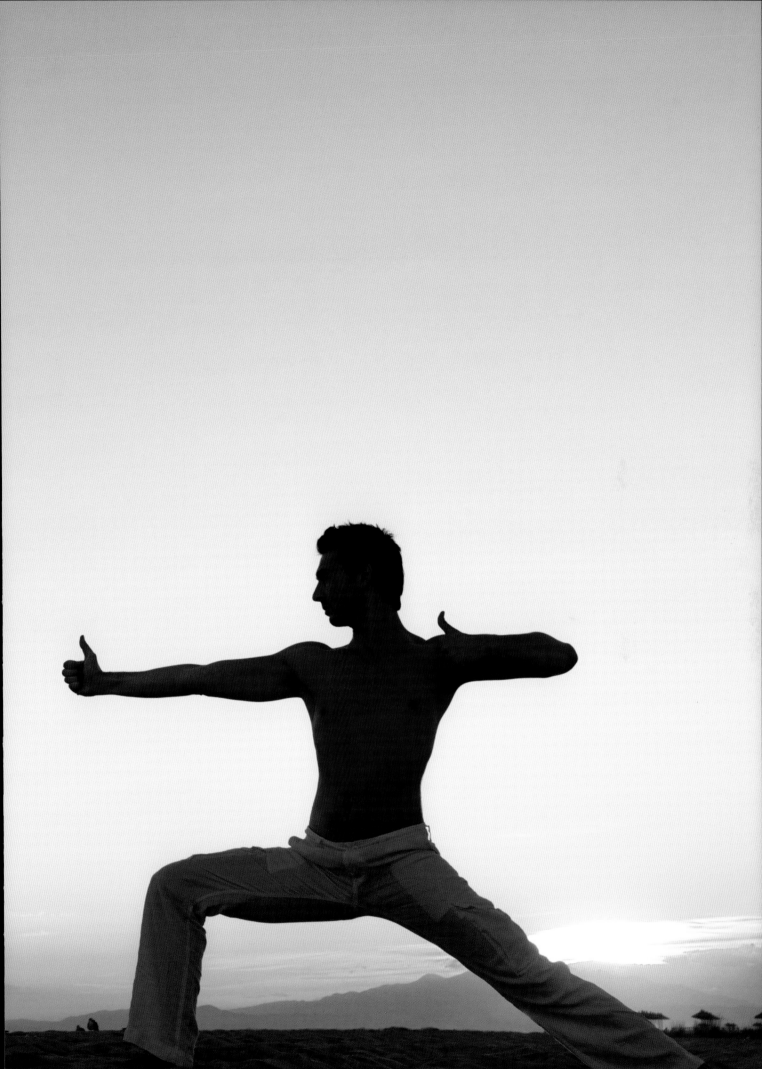

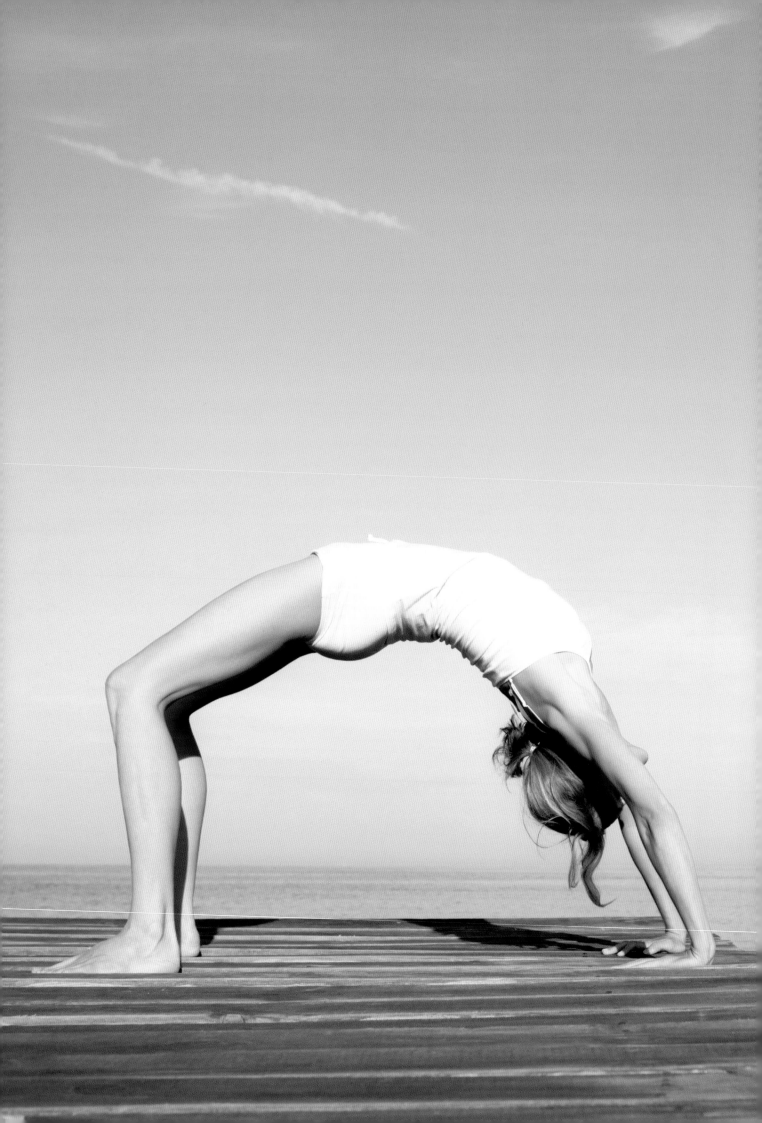

WHEEL POSE

While lying on your back, set your feet hips' width apart and bring them as close as possible to the pelvis. Place the hands next to the head. In this position, your elbows are bent, your forearms are perpendicular to the floor, and your fingers point toward your shoulders. Engage the muscles of your seat and lift the pelvis as high as possible on the inhale. The legs and insides of the feet remain parallel to one another. On the exhale, press yourself higher so that the upper back and shoulders are lifted and only the top of the head touches the floor. On the next inhale, engage mula bandha and press up high into wheel pose by extending the arms and raising the entire body. Shift your weight slightly to your feet. Press the tailbone toward the knees and the pubic bone toward the navel. Relax the head and neck and make sure that the lower back is not being compressed during the exercise.

The wheel position promotes physical flexibility to a higher degree. The thighs, stomach, chest, and shoulders experience a full expansion, and so do the internal organs. The arms, wrists, legs, and the entire back musculature are strengthened, the heart is relaxed, and the pituitary and thyroid glands are stimulated.
This exercise regulates circulation, promotes willpower, and opens the heart center.

BOAT POSE

Lie on your stomach and gaze straight ahead. Stretch your arms over your head and bring your legs together so that the knees, heels, and big toes touch. The palms either face the floor or are together. Engage the musculature of your legs from your seat to your heels. First lift your extended arms and then your legs as high as possible. Ideally, only your stomach will touch the floor. Stretch further, as though you were being stretched by the hands and feet.

The boat pose strengthens the shoulder, spinal, and gluteal musculature and massages the internal organs. This exercise energizes the entire body and supports willpower and resilience.

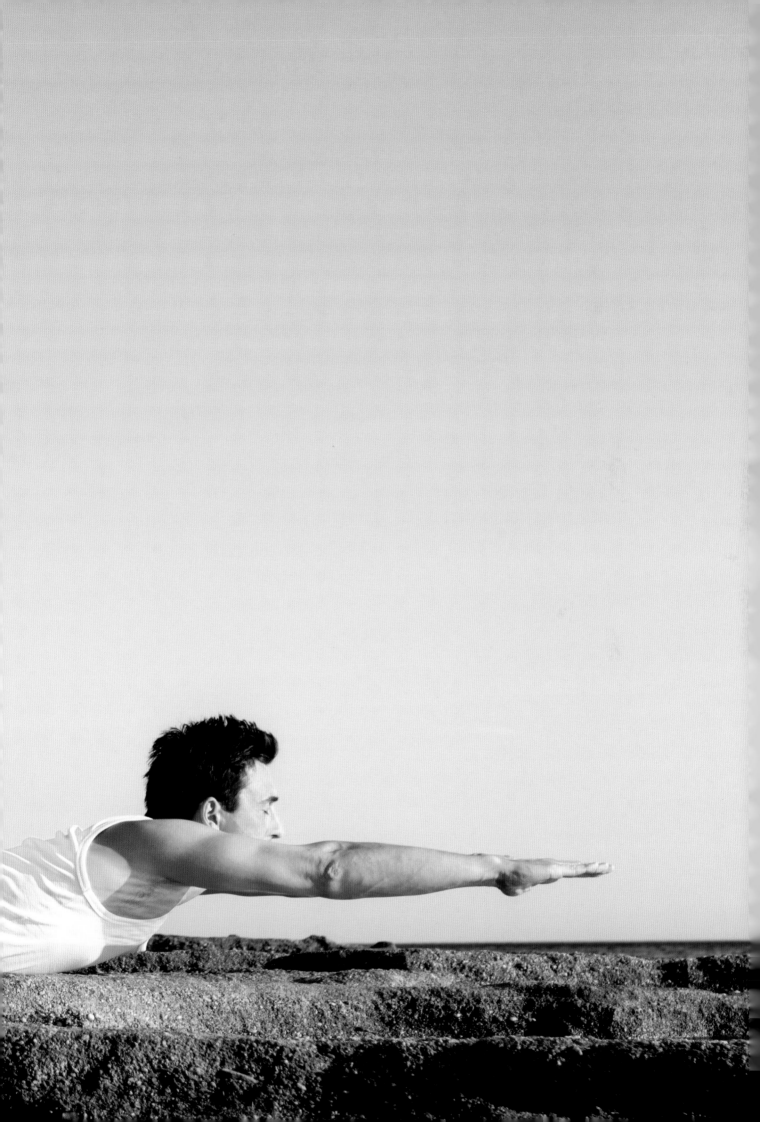

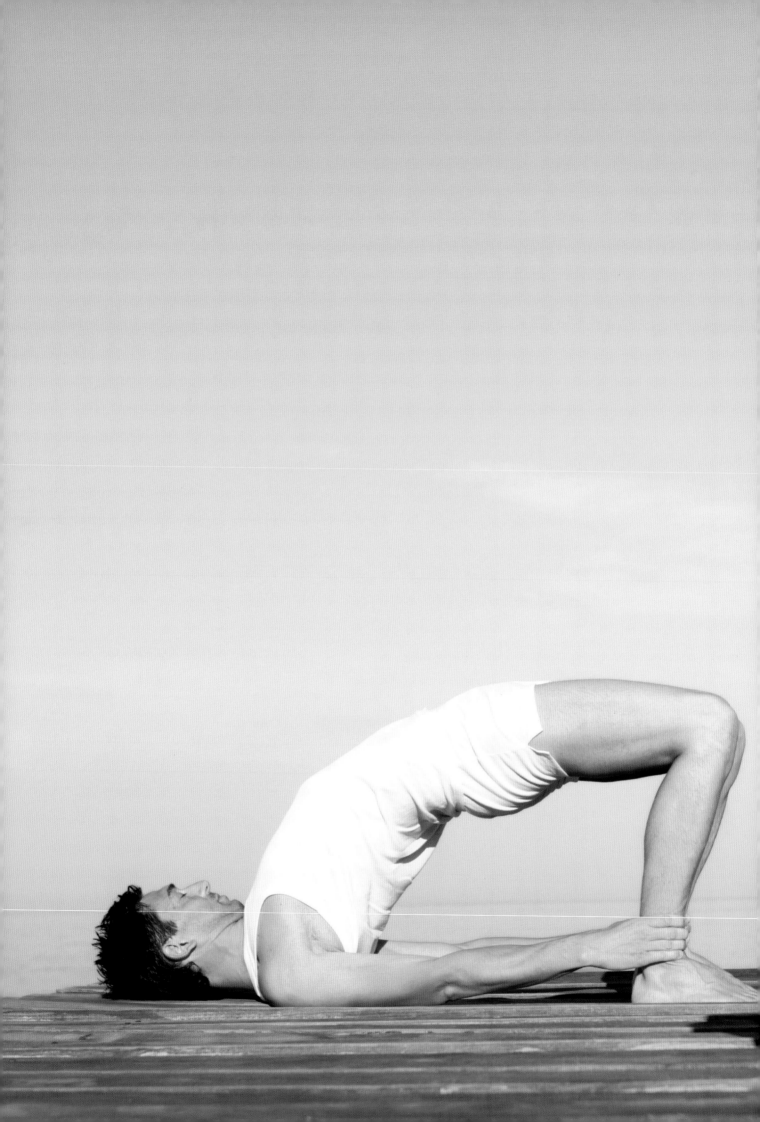

PELVIC LIFTS

While lying on your back, set the feet hips' width apart and bring them as close as possible to the pelvis. Make sure that the soles of the feet remain flat on the floor. Grasp your ankles with your hands. If you cannot reach your ankles, press the palms against the floor next to your hips. Engage the throat lock and mula bandha and begin to lift the pelvis on the inhale. Bring the spine up vertebra by vertebra as far as possible until only the shoulders are touching the floor. Make sure that your lumbar spine is not compressed. Expand the entire chest in this position. On the exhale, come down vertebra by vertebra until finally the pelvis touches the floor again. Repeat the exercise again on the next inhale.

Pelvic lifts strengthen the musculature of the seat and lumbar area, and thus guard against back problems. At the same time, they relaxes the pelvic floor. The energetic connection between the heart, heart, and lower body is improved, stress-related blockages are removed, and desire and creativity are encouraged.

CORPSE POSE

Lie stretched out on your back. The arms lie a slight distance from the body with the palms facing upward and the fingers relaxed. The heels touch and the toes fall loosely to the sides. Close your eyes and breathe in and out slowly and deeply.

In this position, concentrate on your breath, which should be calm and regular, so that the body enters a peaceful state. Now begin to gradually relax each and every muscle in your body. Begin with the toes, calves, knees, and thighs, move over the pelvis, abdomen, and chest to the neck, shoulders, jaw, nose, eyebrows, earlobes, and up to the scalp.

A deep relaxation of about eleven minutes in the corpse pose lets the circulation come to a rest and relieves tension. The body and mind are energetically recharged and endorphin release is activated. This exercise strengthens the immune system and protects against stress-related problems. The energy activated by the asanas is distributed harmoniously through the whole body.

"Self-healing is the privilege of every person. Self-healing is not a miracle and has nothing to do with doing something, being able to do something. Self-healing is a process that develops from the relationship of the body with the infinite power of the soul. It is an engagement, a unity—that is the science of Kundalini Yoga." —Y. B.

KRIYA
KRIYA = ACTION, ACTIVITY

In KUNDALINI YOGA, kriyas are exercise sequences, meditations, or a combination of exercises and meditations. The elements determined by Yogi Bhajan are energetically coordinated and work simultaneously on the body, mind, and soul.

The kriyas differ in regard to length and difficulty. The exercises in a kriya should always be done in the given order and held for the indicated times.

The images in this book serve as guidance. The text instructions are vital to the correct implementation of each exercise.

SAT KRIYA

Come into the kneeling pose and stretch the arms straight up. The fingers are intertwined with only the index fingers pointing straight up. Make sure that the upper arms are next to the ears. Chant the mantra SAT NAM loudly, powerfully, and in an even rhythm (about eight times in ten seconds). On the syllable SAT, pull the navel point in strongly toward the spine. On the syllable NAM, relax the entire belly. Continue for at least three minutes.

Finally, inhale and mentally pull the energy freed by the pumping motion up the entire back from the bottom end of the spinal column. Let it flow up through your crown chakra. You do not need to consciously engage mula bandha, because it happens automatically. Your pose remains unchanged through the entire exercise; only the arms and shoulders move automatically due to the movement of the navel point.

Relaxation following this exercise should last twice as long as the kriya.

Sat kriya is elementary in KUNDALINI YOGA. It should be performed daily and should generally be combined with the mantra SAT NAM.

Sat kriya can be performed for up to thirty-one minutes. However, the length should be increased only gradually, because the kriya affects all levels of the being, both unconsciously and consciously. The body should be prepared slowly for the rising energies, because otherwise the developing experience of consciousness cannot be fully incorporated into the psyche. To increase the duration of the exercise, it is recommended that you practice the kriya for three minutes and rest for two minutes. This cycle should be repeated until you reach fifteen minutes of sat kriya and ten minutes of rest. A twenty-minute rest should follow at the end.

Sat kriya can also be practiced with the palms flat together. In this case, more energy will be released than in the variation described above. Therefore it is important that the body is completely free of drugs (for example, narcotics, caffeine, nicotine) and in the case of earlier consumption, also cleansed of their effects.

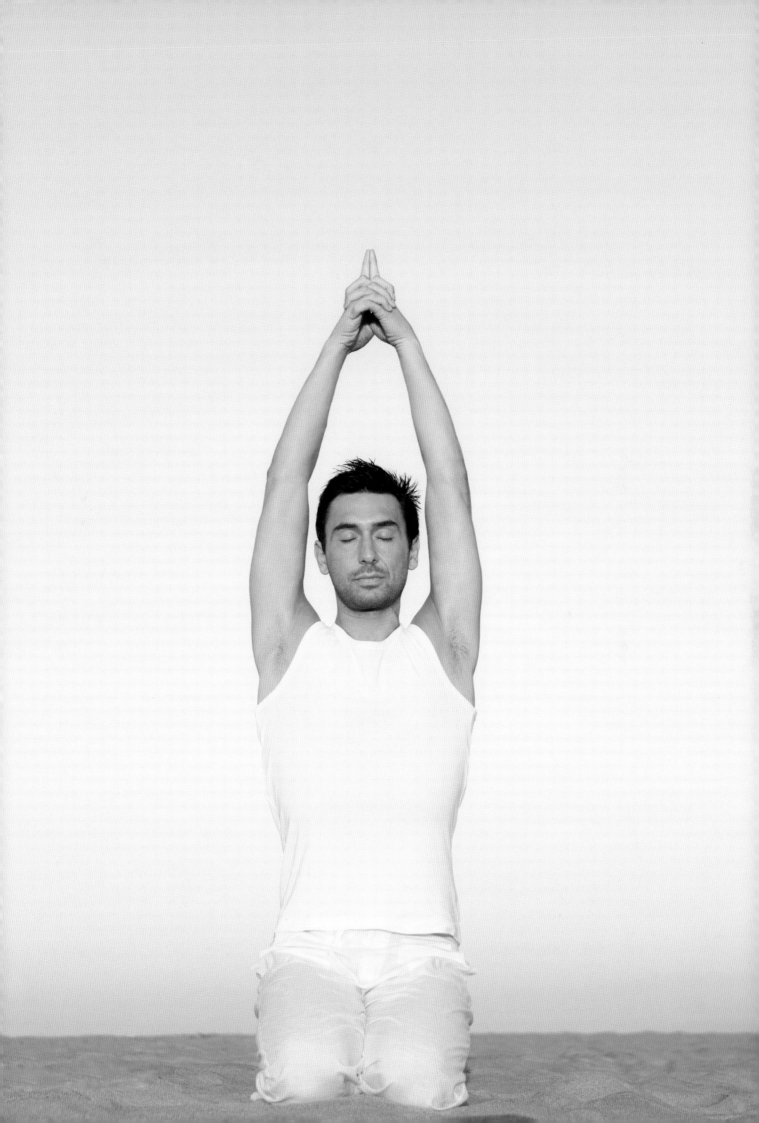

VARUYAS KRIYA

Stand up straight with your legs together. Take a small step forward with your right foot and step back into a wide lunge with your left foot. Place your left foot on the floor, or, to intensify the effect, lay the top of your foot on the floor. Make sure that your right knee is positioned vertically above your ankle. Stretch your arms forward horizontally and press your palms together. Tilt your upper body forward slightly and direct your gaze to a point on the horizon or concentrate on the third eye. Engage mula bandha, inhale deeply, and begin to sing SAT NAM rhythmically. With each SAT, pull the navel point toward the spinal column, and relax your entire abdomen with each NAM. Finally, inhale and exhale deeply and relax. Then switch leg positions and repeat the exercise. Time: 1½–7½ minutes

Varuyas Kriya can be performed as an individual exercise or in connection with a series which stimulates the circulation or promotes flexibility.

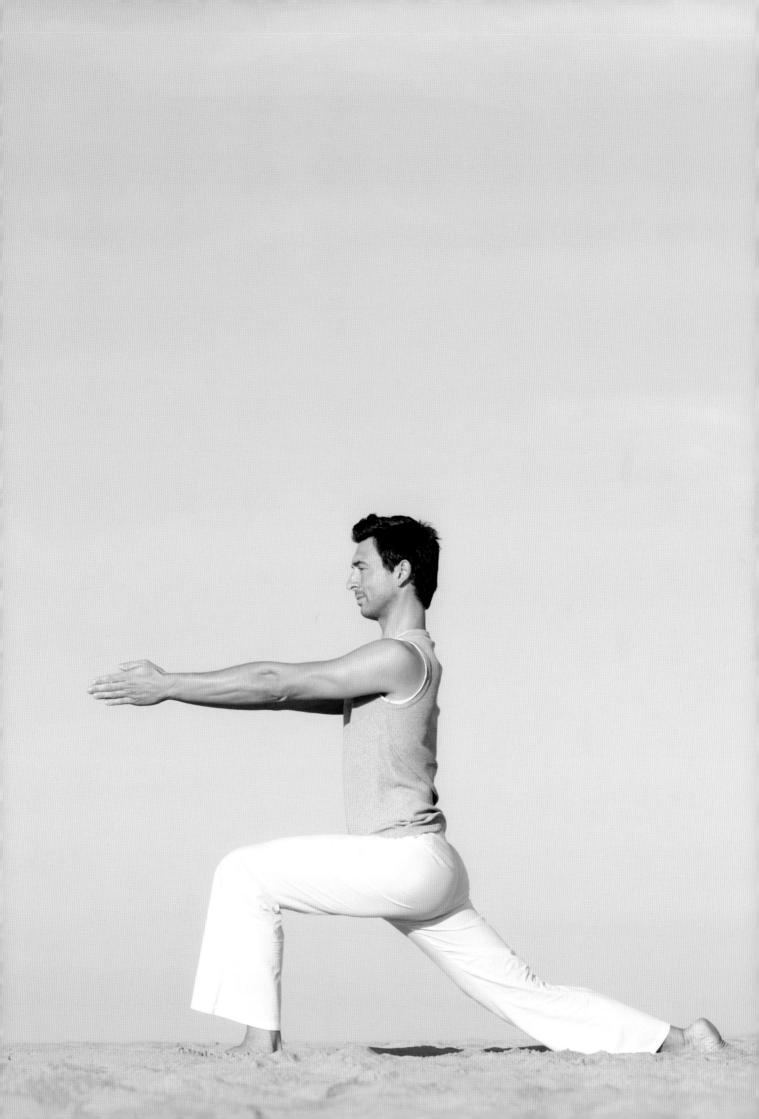

WAKE-UP SERIES

1 While lying on your back, stretch your arms and legs, raise your head slightly, and look toward your toes. Lift your arms and legs six inches (fifteen centimeters) from the floor and begin the breath of fire. Your fingertips should point toward your toes. Finally, inhale and exhale deeply and release the pose. If you cannot hold the pose for more than a minute, release the pose, relax, and then begin again.
Time: 1–2 minutes
Connects Prana with Apana.

2 While lying on your back, bend your legs, bring your knees to your chest, and grasp them in your arms. Lift your head until your nose is between your knees and begin the breath of fire. Finally, inhale and exhale deeply and release the pose. Time: 2 minutes
This exercise positions the navel point.

3 While lying on your back, grasp your bent knees with your hands. On the exhale, roll forward on your spine, and on the exhale, roll back. Time: 1 minute
Distributes the Prana energy and relaxes the spine.

4 In the simple seated pose, lift your extended arms up to the sides so that they each form a 60° angle to the floor. The fingertips touch the base of the fingers and the thumbs are extended and point up vertically. Breathe the breath of fire for two minutes. Conclude the exercise by lifting your arms up very slowly until your thumbs touch above your head. Lower your arms while you exhale with palms facing downward. Cleanse and strengthen your aura by collecting all negative energy in your hands and releasing it through the palms into the earth.

Yogi Bhajan advises practicing this series in bed daily before rising.

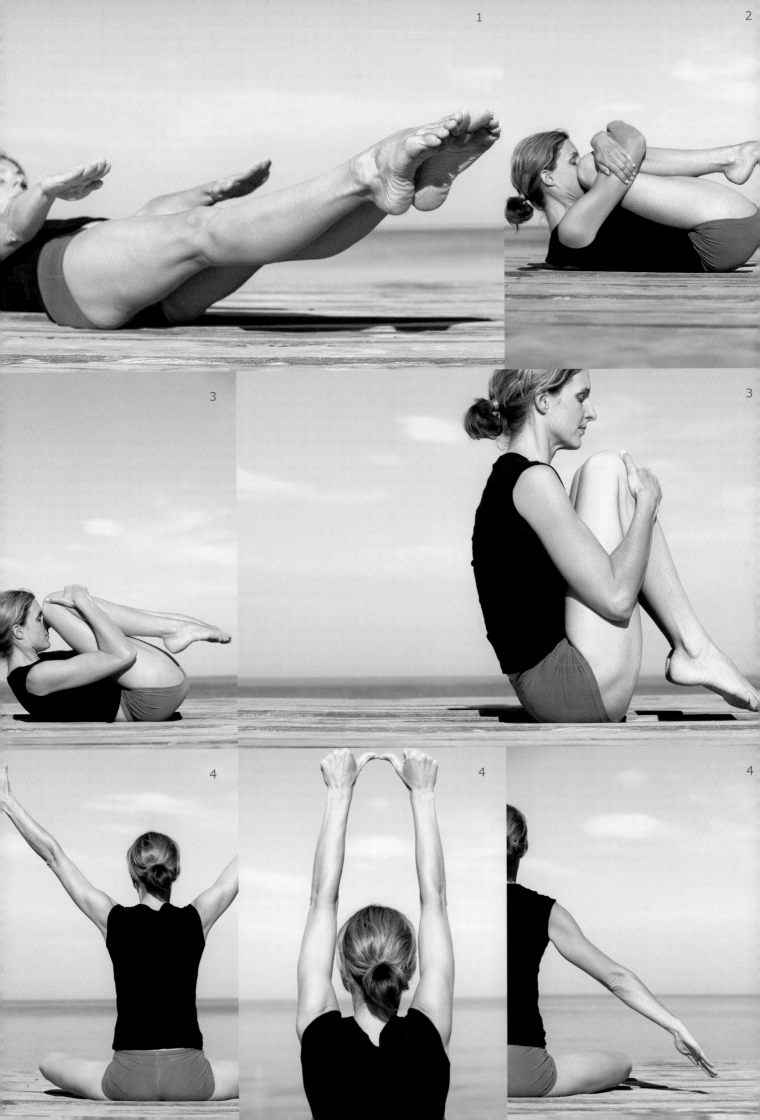

ACTIVATING THE KUNDALINI ENERGY

1 Place your feet shoulder width apart and lower into a squat. Bring your arms between the insides of your thighs to the outsides of your calves and grasp the outsides of your feet with your hands. Your spine is straight and parallel to the floor. Your breath is long and deep. Finally, inhale and exhale deeply and hold the exhale while engaging mula bandha. Release the pose and relax. Time: 2–3 minutes

2 In the simple seated pose, grasp the shins. Inhale and pull your upper body up vertically. Relax the pose on the exhale but remain sitting upright. Make sure that your upper body tilts neither forward nor backward. Finally, inhale and exhale deeply and hold the exhale while engaging mula bandha. Release the pose and relax. Time: 2–3 minutes

3 In the simple seated pose, do torso twists. Let the mantra SAT resonate in your mind with each inhale and with each exhale the mantra NAM. Align yourself facing forward on the last repetition, hold your breath briefly, and release the pose on the exhale. Time: 2–3 minutes

4 In the simple seated pose, stretch your arms up vertically, press the palms together, and continue with torso twists. Align yourself facing forward on the last repetition, inhale and exhale deeply, and hold the exhale while engaging mula bandha. Release the pose and relax. Time: 2–3 minutes

5 While seated, stretch out your legs and place your hands next to your hips. If you cannot reach the floor with your hands, make them into fists. If you are experienced, you can also go into the lotus position. Inhale and push yourself up vertically with your hands until your seat is lifted from the floor. Let yourself sink back down on the exhale. Make sure that your spinal column remains straight during the entire exercise. Finally, inhale and exhale deeply and hold the exhale while engaging mula bandha. Release the pose and relax. Time: 2–3 minutes

6 Sit with outstretched legs. Bend as far forward as is possible for you. Ideally, you will grasp your feet in your hands and touch your knees with your forehead. Relax in this pose. Finally, inhale and exhale deeply and hold the exhale while engaging mula bandha. Release the pose and relax. Time: 2–3 minutes

7 Continue to sit upright and leave your legs outstretched. Cross your extended arms in front of your chest. Touch your right knee with your left hand and your left knee with your right hand. Inhale deeply, hold your breath, and extend the arms and shoulders. Then release the pose and relax.

8 In the simple seated pose, bring your hands in front of your chest and hook your index fingers together. Now pull your arms apart strongly without losing your grip. Take long, slow breaths. Finally, inhale deeply, reach your arms over your head, exhale and engage mula bandha. Release the pose and relax. Time: 2–3 minutes

9 Pull yourself into bow from a prone position and begin taking long, deep breaths. Finally, inhale, hold the inhale while engaging mula bandha, hold for a moment, and then breathe out. Release the pose and relax. Time: 2–3 minutes

10 For the closing meditation, go into the simple seated pose again. The hands are in the ghyan mudra and your attention is on the crown of your head. Press your tongue up against your palate, which may cause a slight pain in your nose. Join with your Higher Self.

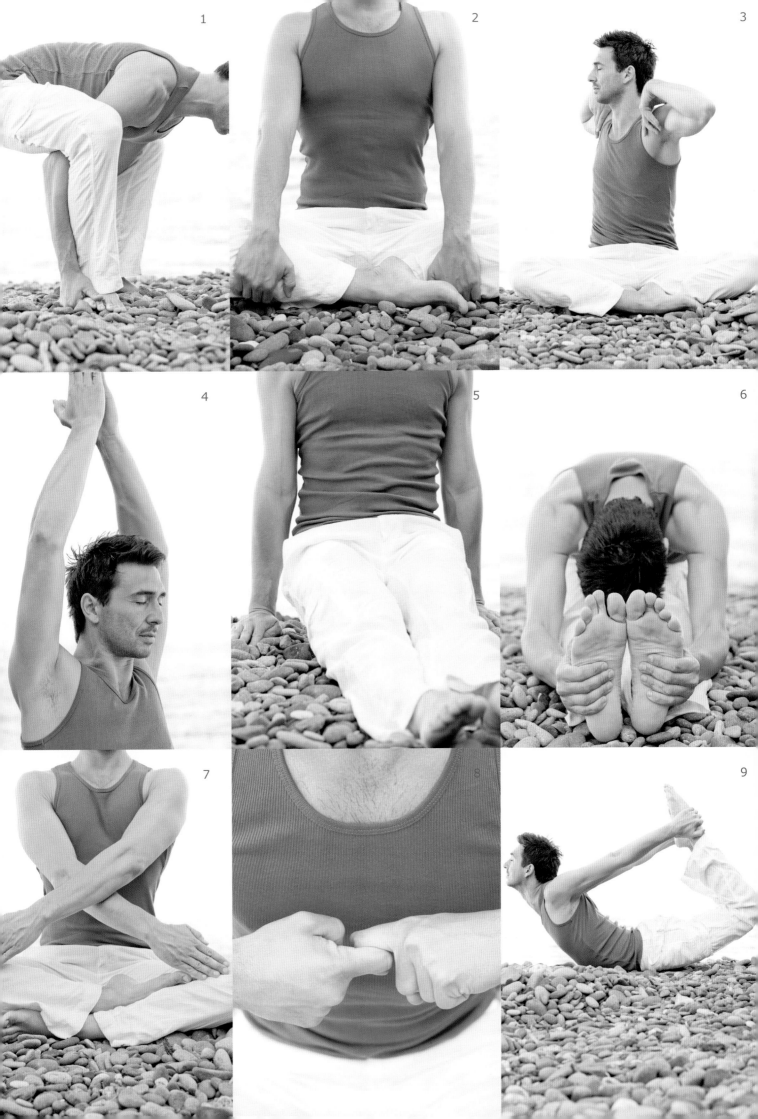

BASIC SPINAL ENERGY SERIES

1 In the simple seated pose, grasp the ankles with the hands and begin the camel ride. With each inhale think SAT and with each exhale think NAM. Make sure that you keep the head straight. Finally, inhale and exhale deeply, release the pose, and relax for one minute. Repetitions: 108

2 In the kneeling pose, place the hands flat on the thighs and repeat the camel ride. Let SAT vibrate through your mind with each inhale and NAM with each exhale. Finally, inhale and exhale deeply, release the pose, and relax for two minutes. Repetitions: 108 (not depicted)

3 Lay the hands on the shoulders, thumbs pointing backward, fingers forward. In the simple seated pose, begin spinal twists. With each inhale think SAT and with each exhale think NAM. Finally, inhale and exhale deeply, release the pose, and relax for one minute. Repetitions: 26

4 Stay in the simple seated pose and hook the hands in front of the chest in the bear grip. Begin with the long deep breath and rock the elbows alternately up and down. Lift the left elbow on the inhale and the right on the exhale. Make sure that your forearms always create a line. Finally, inhale and exhale deeply and pull the arms apart powerfully. Exhale, release your arm position, and relax for thirty seconds. Repetitions: 26

5 In the simple seated pose, grasp your knees. Like in the camel ride, bend your thoracic spine forward on the exhale and back on the inhale. Let SAT vibrate through your mind with each inhale and NAM with each exhale. The arms remain extended the entire time. Finally, inhale and exhale deeply in an upright seated position, release the pose, and relax for one minute.

6 Remain in the simple seated pose. Pull the shoulders up to the ears on the inhale and let them fall back down loosely on the exhale. Repeat this motion. Finally, inhale deeply with shoulders lifted high. Hold your breath for fifteen seconds. Release the pose on the exhale and relax. Length: up to 2 minutes

7 In the simple seated pose, roll your head first five times clockwise and then five times counterclockwise. Finally, inhale deeply, engage the throat lock while holding the inhale, release the pose on the exhale and relax.

8 In the simple seated pose, fold the hands into the bear grip. On the inhale, lift the arms over the head and let them sink back in front of the chest on the exhale. Engage mula bandha on the inhale and the exhale. Finally, inhale and exhale deeply, release the pose, and relax. Repetitions: 2

9 In the kneeling pose, stretch the arms straight up and begin sat kriya. Inhale and mentally pull the energy from the bottom of your spine up to the crown. Release the pose on the exhale and relax. Length: at least 3 minutes

10 Lie on your back and relax. Length: 15 minutes

If you have less experience, you can reduce the repetition from 108 to 26 and stretch the relaxing pauses to two minutes.

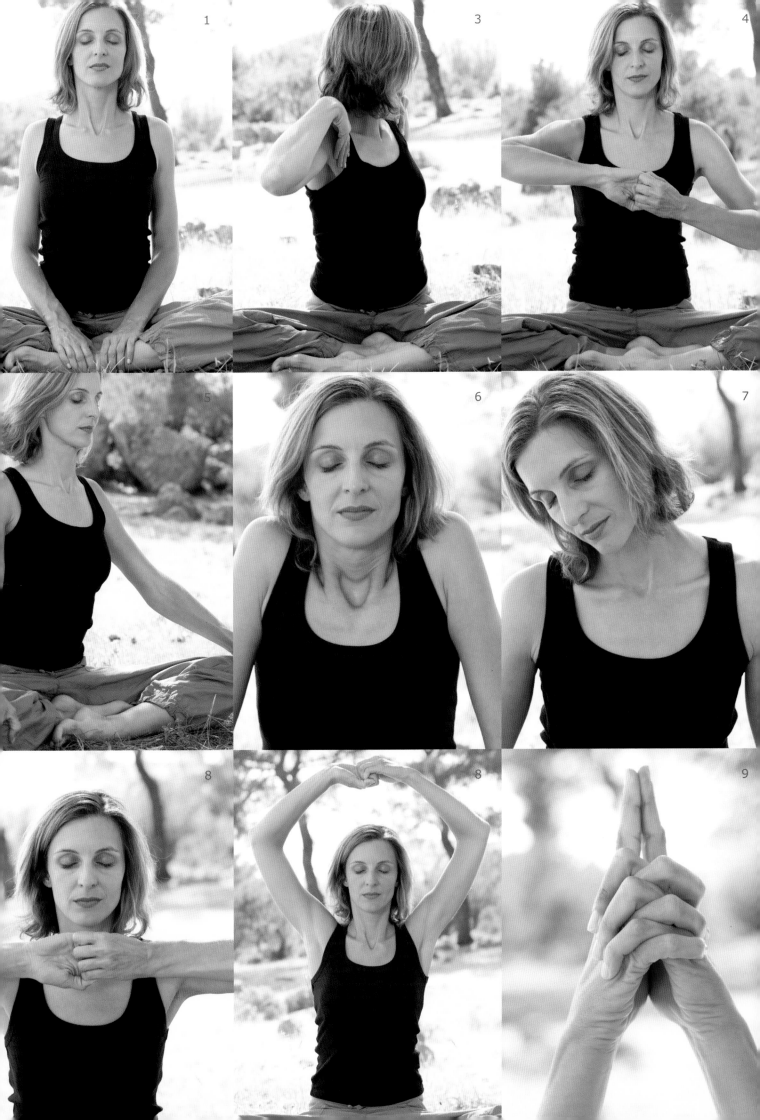

KRIYA FOR STRENGTHENING DISEASE RESISTANCE

1 In the kneeling position, stretch the arms over the head and press the palms together. Inhale, hold your breath, and powerfully move the belly in and out toward the spine as many times as possible in a steady rhythm. Exhale and, with the next inhale, begin the pumping motion again. Finally, inhale and exhale deeply, release the pose, and relax. Length: 1-3 minutes
Activates digestion and stimulates the Kundalini energy in the third chakra.

2 Fold the hands into the bear grip in front of the chest. Breathe in, hold your breath, and pull the hands apart as firmly as possible without losing your grip. Exhale and loosen the grip. Repeat the exercise with the next inhale. Finally, inhale and exhale deeply, release the pose, and relax. Length: 1-3 minutes
Opens the heart chakra and stimulates the thymus gland.

3 Interlace the fingers behind the neck in the Venus grip. Inhale and bend forward with a straight back until the forehead touches the floor. Rise again on the inhale. Repeat the cycle with powerful breaths. Finally, inhale and exhale deeply, release the pose, and relax. Length: 1-3 minutes
Improves digestion and increases flexibility of the spine.

4 Sit with outstretched legs and bend your upper body over them, keeping your back straight. Try to grasp your big toes with your index and middle fingers and lay your forehead on your knees. Make sure that the legs remain extended. Stay in this position, breathing normally. Finally, inhale and exhale deeply, release the pose, and relax. Length: 1-2 minutes
Helps the body relax more deeply.

5 In the simple seated pose, roll your head clockwise. Halfway through the time, change the direction. Finally, inhale and exhale deeply, release the pose, and relax. Length: 2-4 minutes each direction

6 Come to your hands and knees to begin cat-cow. Gradually raise the speed. Your breath is deep and powerful the entire time. Finally, inhale and exhale deeply in the cow position, release the pose, and relax. Length: 1-3 minutes
Helps to transform the sexual energy and the energy in the digestive tract.

7 While in the kneeling pose, raise the shoulders alternately to the ears without moving the head. Lift the left shoulder on the inhale and the right shoulder on the exhale. Repeat with powerful breath. Finally, inhale, raise both shoulders high, exhale, release the pose, and relax. Length: 1-3 minutes
Exercises 5-7 increase blood flow to the brain and stimulate the glandular system.

8 Lie on your back and relax. Length: 5-7 minutes

9 Come into downward dog and stay there. Breathe naturally. Finally, inhale and exhale deeply, release the pose, and relax.
Improves digestion, strengthens the entire nervous system, and relaxes the major muscle groups.

10 Stand up, bend forward as far as possible, and grasp your ankles. Make sure that your knees are extended. Take small steps around the room in this position. Finally, stand up and relax. Length: 1-3 minutes
Supports digestion and prepares the aura for meditation.

11 Lie on your back and relax.

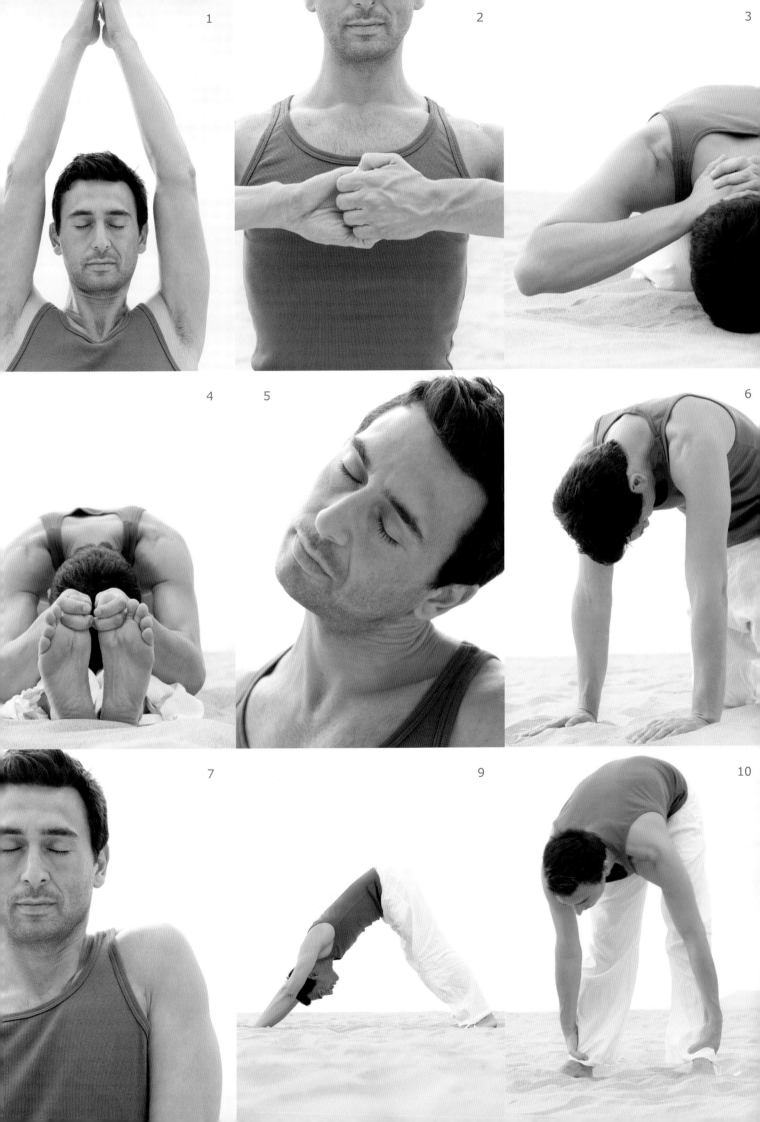

KRIYA FOR OVERCOMING INSOMNIA

1 In the kneeling pose, gently lay the palms on the thighs. Lean back with your entire spine until your torso creates a 60° angle to the floor. Your breath is long and deep. Finally, inhale and exhale deeply, release the pose, and relax. Length: 1 minute

2 Cross your arms in front of your chest, grasping the elbows. Move your torso clockwise in a circle. Make sure that your back remains straight. Finally, sit up straight, inhale and exhale deeply, release the pose, and relax. Length: 3 minutes

3 Sit with outstretched legs and place your hands next to your hips. Make fists if you cannot reach the ground. On the inhale, press yourself up so that the seat and, if possible, also the thighs are lifted from the floor. On the exhale, let yourself sink back into the starting position. Repeat the cycle. Finally, inhale and exhale deeply, release the pose, and relax. Repetitions: 20

4 Repeat exercise 2. Length: 3 minutes

5 Repeat exercise 3. Repetitions: 15

6 Sit down, bend your knees, place your feet in front of you, and support yourself on your hands as you lean back. Lift the pelvis and come into the bridge pose. Make sure that the calves and arms stand perpendicular to the floor. The knees, pelvis, and shoulders create a line parallel to the floor. Let the head relax back from the neck and breathe slowly and deeply for one minute. Continue the exercise with the breath of fire. Three minutes. To finish, exhale fully and engage mula bandha while holding the exhale. Finally, release the pose and relax.

7 Repeat exercise 3. Repetitions: 10

8 Repeat exercise 6 and breathe the breath of fire. Finally, exhale completely and engage mula bandha while holding the exhale. Release the pose and relax. Length: 3 minutes

9 Lie on your back and relax. Length: 2-3 minutes

10 Return to the bridge pose and lift the right leg so that it creates a 60° angle to the floor. Stretch the toes forward. Let the head relax back from the neck. Begin the breath of fire in this position. Finally, exhale fully and engage mula bandha while holding the exhale. Repeat the exercise with the left leg outstretched. Release the pose and relax. Length: 1½ minutes per side

11 Squat with the torso upright and the feet flat on the floor. Stretch the arms straight out ahead of you with palms facing downward. On the inhale stand straight up, and on the exhale squat back down. Make sure that the spine remains as straight as possible during the entire exercise. Repetitions: 30

12 Lift yourself into cobra pose from a prone position. Breathe long and deep for one minute. Then on each exhale begin to kick against your seat with your left heel. After one minute, switch to the other side and kick with your right heel. Finally, inhale and exhale deeply, release the pose, and relax.

13 In the kneeling pose, lift slightly bent arms overhead and press the palms together. Engage the throat lock and concentrate on the crown of your head and on the pineal gland. Imagine you are looking up through your cranium. Length: at least 3 minutes

This kriya helps with insomnia and should be practiced for ninety days, either in the morning after waking or in the evening before going to sleep.

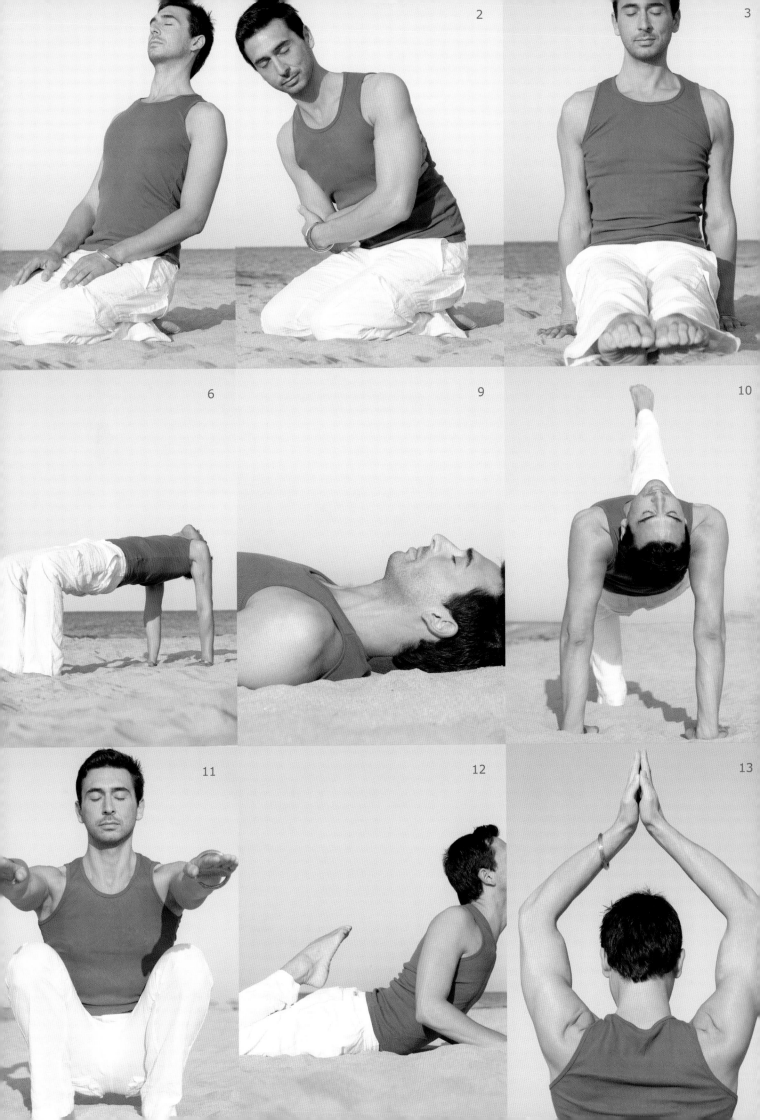

EXERCISE SERIES FOR THE KIDNEYS

1 Sit with outstretched legs and lift the arms straight ahead. The fingertips touch the bases of the fingers and the thumbs are stretched straight up. Inhale and exhale, and on the exhale bend as far forward as possible with a straight back. Make sure that the arms remain parallel to the floor. The breath becomes deeper and more powerful during the exercise. Finally, inhale and exhale deeply, release the pose, and relax. Length: 5-6 minutes

2 Begin with pelvis lifts. Lift on the inhale, lower on the exhale. Finally, inhale and exhale deeply, release the pose, and relax. Length: 8 minutes
Strengthens the neck, stimulates the kidneys and bladder, and is helpful with hernia. The powerful breath stimulates the pituitary gland.

3a Begin with cat-cow. Inhale when you lift the head and exhale when you lower it. Continuously increase the speed. Finally, inhale deeply in the cow pose. Length: 2 minutes

3b In the cow pose, stretch the left leg out horizontally and hold it in this position. After thirty seconds, change to the other leg. Length: 30 seconds each

3c Lift the left leg straight out again in the cow pose. Kick with the left foot against the left side of the seat. After one minute, inhale and exhale deeply, switch and kick for thirty seconds with the right heel against the right half of the seat. Finally, inhale and exhale deeply and release the pose.
Exercise 3 improves kidney function.

4 Lie on your back and bend your knees to your chest, embracing your legs. Lift your head so that you can hold your nose between your knees. Relax for one to two minutes in this position. Finally, sing the song "Nobility" (p. 142) for five to six minutes and "Everything comes from God and everything returns to God" for two minutes in the same position. Alternatively, you can breathe long and deep for seven to nine minutes.

5a Squat and stretch the arms straight out. The feet are flat on the floor, the back is straight, and the palms face downward. Remain in this position. Length: 2-3 minutes

5b Begin to continuously chant the mantra HAR HAR HAR in this position. Make sure that the tongue touches the gums right behind the front teeth during this mantra. Length: 2-3 minutes

5c Remain in this position and engage the musculature of the mouth and lips on the inhale. Hold your breath for twenty seconds and concentrate on posture. Exhale and inhale again. This time, hold your breath for thirty seconds, engage the mouth and lip musculature again, and concentrate all your attention on your balance. Finally, inhale and exhale deeply, release the pose, and relax.
Stimulates the kidneys and urinary tract. If you feel slightly dizzy during the exercise, it is a sign that your body needs more water.

6a In the simple seated pose, put the hands in ghyan mudra. Stretch the arms straight ahead with palms facing down. Bend your left arm so that the fingertips point to the right elbow. Now angle the right forearm up and bend the hand back so the back of the hand is parallel to the upper arm. Accuracy is essential in this mudra. Stretch the spine. Pull the navel in and the ribcage up. Engage the muscles of the seat and pelvis and pull yourself up until you don't feel any more weight on the sitz bones. Relax after thirty seconds. Continue engaging and relaxing. During the entire exercise, engage the throat lock. Finally, inhale and exhale deeply and relax. Length: 5 minutes

6b Hold the above muscle tension and sing the mantra WAHE GURU WAHE GURU WAHE JIO. Concentrate on your breath at the same time. The eyelids become heavy and the breath becomes lighter and lighter. Finally, inhale and exhale deeply, release the pose, and relax. Length: 5 minutes
This exercise has a strongly relaxing and cleansing effect on the entire body. There is no time limit for this position; the length of the exercise should, however, be built up slowly and continuously.

7 Relax deeply for a long time.

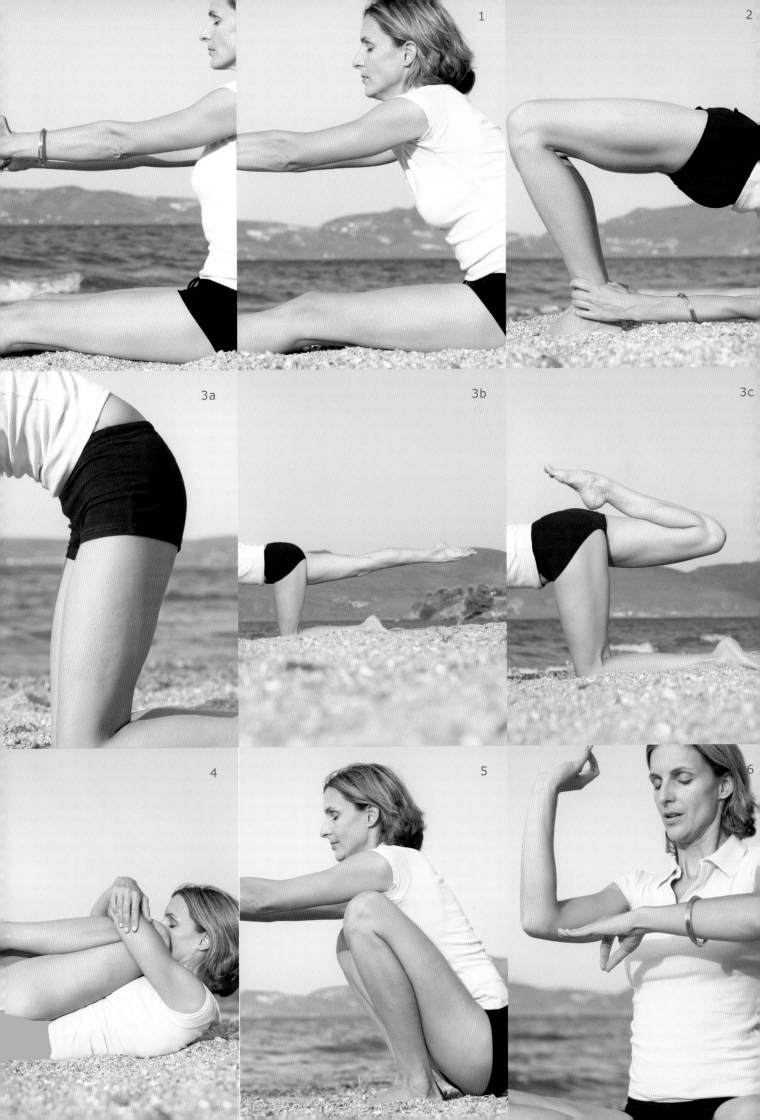

1

2

3a

3b

3c

4

5

6

NEW OPPORTUNITIES AND GREEN ENERGY

1 Sit in the kneeling pose and begin the camel ride. Think SAT on the inhale and concentrate on the first chakra; think NAM on the exhale and direct your attention to the fourth chakra.
Length: 2–3 minutes
To finish, sit up straight. Inhale deeply and hold the inhale, engage mula bandha, exhale and hold the exhale, and engage mula bandha for ten more seconds. Repeat this three times. Release the pose and relax.

2 Sit with your legs outstretched and place your hands next to your hips. Make fists if you cannot reach the floor. On the inhale, push up with your arms so that your seat lifts up from the floor. On the exhale, let yourself sink carefully back to the original position. Make sure that your back remains straight through the entire exercise. Repeat the cycle. Finally, inhale and exhale deeply, release the pose, and relax.
Length: 2-3 minutes

3 Squat with feet flat on the floor. Stretch the arms straight ahead and interlace the hands in the Venus lock with the index fingers stretched out pointing forward. Make sure that the spine remains as straight and upright as possible. Begin the breath of fire. Finally, inhale and exhale deeply, release the pose, and relax. Length: 2-3 minutes

4 Stand upright. Begin to run vigorously in place. Lift the knees strongly and make boxing motions with your fists. Length: 3-5 minutes

5 Sit in the Kundalini lotus position and begin the breath of fire. Finally, inhale, hold the inhale, pull the energy up along the entire spine, and exhale. Releases the pose and relax. Length: 2-3 minutes

6 Sit on the right foot and lay the left foot on the right thigh. The hands lie together in the lap and the tips of the thumbs touch. Lift the diaphragm, sing ONG SO HANG loudly and powerfully, and listen to the sound of the mantra with your heart. Finally, inhale and exhale deeply, release the pose, and relax.

7 In the simple seated pose, stretch the arms straight out to the sides with the palms facing upward. Concentrate on how the energy from your left hand flows in a large bow over your head into your right hand and from your right hand through your arms and shoulders back to the left hand. Feel this strong bow between your hands. Begin the breath of fire. Finally, inhale, hold the inhale, and feel the further flowing of the energy. Exhale, release the pose, and relax. Length: 2-3 minutes ▶ ▶

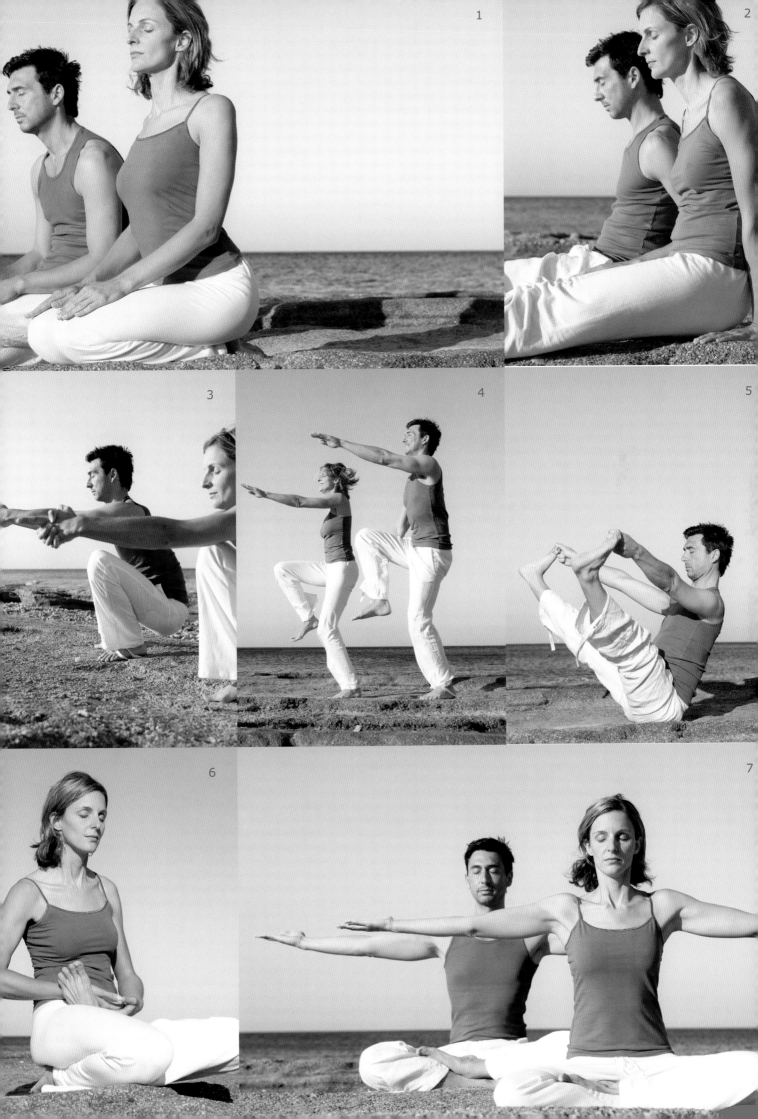

8 Remain in the simple seated pose and interlace the hands behind the neck in the Venus lock. Exhale, think SAT, and bend until your forehead touches the floor. Think NAM on the exhale and come back to the original upright position. Finally, inhale and exhale deeply, release the pose, and relax. Length: 2-3 minutes

9 In the simple seated pose, stretch your arms straight ahead with palms facing downward. On the inhale, lift the right arm up so that it creates a 60° angle with the floor. Lower the arm back to the starting position on the exhale and, at the same time, lift the left arm. Repeat this exercise without pausing. The breath is like the breath of fire. Then lift both arms to the height of your third eye. Inhale, hold your breath and direct your attention out from your third eye into infinity. Exhale, release the pose, and relax. Length: 2-3 minutes

10a In the simple seated pose, interlace your fingers in the Venus lock and lift your hands about four inches above your head. The palms face upward. Direct your attention above yourself through the crown chakra and begin the breath of fire. Length: 2-3 minutes

10b In the same position, stretch your index fingers up and press them together. Continue to concentrate up through the seventh chakra. Now breathe long and deep. Length: 2-3 minutes

10c Remain in the same position. Put the fingertips together to create a pyramid over your head. Your concentration should still be directed at the crown and, from there, farther up. Begin the breath of fire. Finally, inhale and hold the inhale with your attention still directed up. Exhale, release the pose, and relax. Length: 2-3 minutes

11a In the simple seated pose, pull your upper arms close to your body. Angle your forearms up vertically. The hands are extended and the palms face forward. Visualize green light and green energy, pull in your navel point gently, and chant HARI HARI HARI HARI from your heart. Finally, inhale and exhale deeply and relax in ghyan mudra. Length: 2-11 minutes

11b In the simple seated pose, meditate and contemplate all the things that you can be thankful for. Feel yourself in the middle of a rain of clean energy. Enjoy every single breath and send your love to all-that-is.

12 Lie on your back and relax.

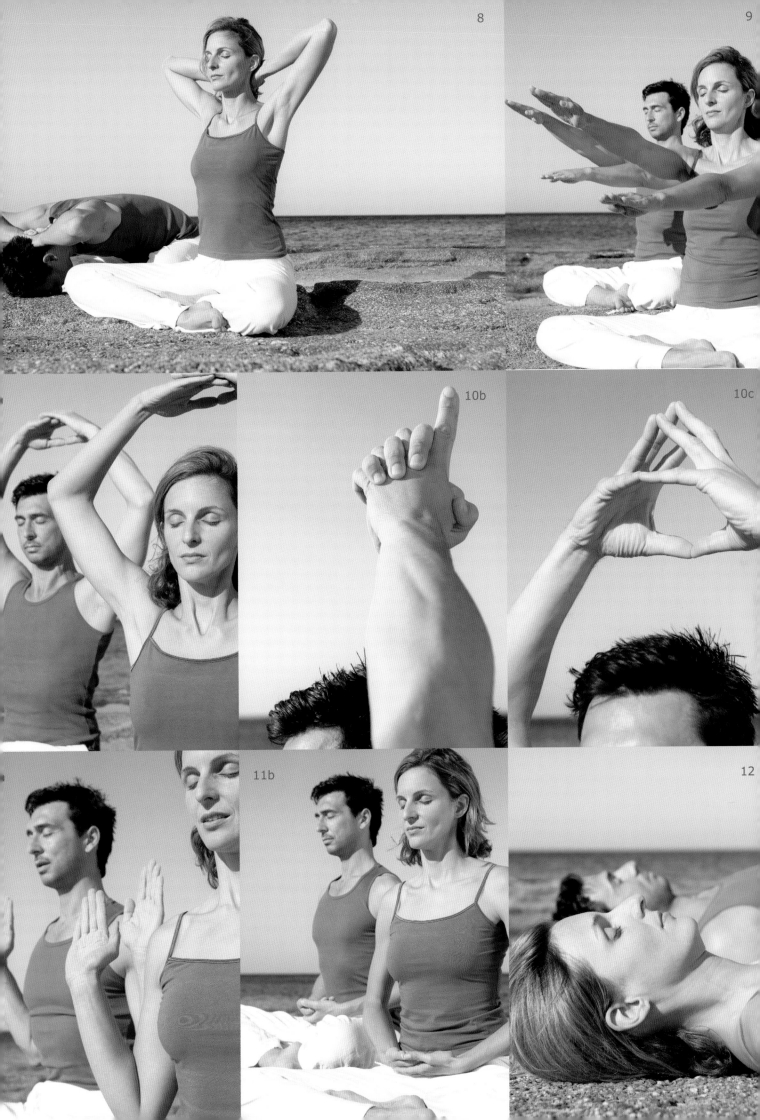

CLEANSING SERIES FOR BEGINNERS

1 Lie on your back and interlace your fingers behind your neck in the Venus lock. Breathe the breath of fire for a minute and a half. Inhale and hold for twenty seconds. Repeat the breath of fire, inhale, and hold for thirty seconds. Exhale and let the breath become calmer. Inhale, hold the inhale, and lift the legs off the floor for fifteen seconds. Lower the legs on the exhale and relax.
Activates pulmonary circulation and the energy of the navel point.

2 Lie on your back and spread your legs apart. Breathe the breath of fire for one minute, inhale deeply, and lift the legs about thirty-five inches from the floor for five seconds. Let them come down to the floor on the exhale, still spread. Repeat the breath of fire and lift the legs four more times. On the last cycle, lift the legs twelve inches and hold them up as long as possible while holding the inhale. Finally, exhale, lower the legs, and relax.
Exercises 2 and 3 activate the sexual energy.

3 Bring the legs together, still lying on your back, so that the knees and heels touch. Lift the feet, the extended arms, and the head six inches from the floor and gaze toward the heels. Begin the breath of fire. Finally, inhale deeply, release the pose on the exhale, and relax. Length: 3 minutes
This exercise activates the navel point.

4 Sit upright and stretch the legs out forward. Lay the left foot on the right thigh, so that the sole of the foot faces upward. Stretch the arms out straight in front of you until the hands are next to the right foot. Grasp the toes. On the inhale lean back so that your straight back creates a 60° angle with the floor. Repeat this cycle twenty-five times. Finally, stretch out the opposite leg and repeat the exercise another twenty-five times.
Strengthens the lower spine and regulates chemical balance in the blood.

5a Remain sitting upright with outstretched legs. Lean back again at 60° and support yourself on extended arms at shoulders' width. Lean the head back carefully, look up and fix your gaze on one point. Try not to blink and breathe the breath of fire for two minutes.

5b Inhale in the same position, hold the inhale, and lift the legs twelve inches off the floor for fifteen to twenty seconds. Lower the legs on the exhale.

5c Remain in the same position and breathe the breath of fire for one minute. Inhale deeply, hold the inhale, and lift the legs twelve inches off the floor for fifteen seconds. Lower the legs on the exhale and relax on your back.
This exercise brings energy to the eyes and brain. Proven to work for headache and eye illness.

6 Lie on your back and inhale deeply, then exhale completely. Hold the exhale and lift extended arms straight up. Make fists and bring them slowly to your chest. Engage the arms strongly, as though you were pushing against resistance. The fists will begin to shake automatically when they touch the chest. Inhale and exhale several times and repeat the exercise while holding the inhale.
Eliminates remaining tension.

7 Lie on your back and relax. Length: 5 minutes

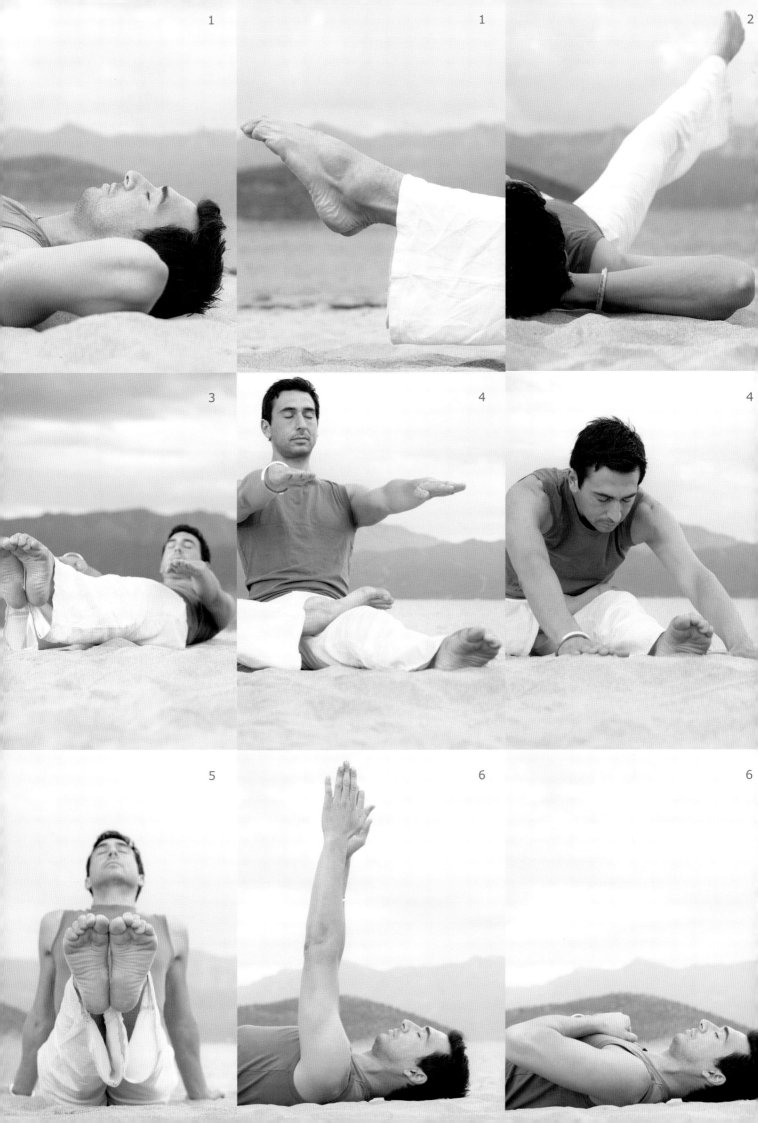

SURYA KRIYA

1 In the simple seated pose, lay the right hand on the right knee in gyan mudra. Close the left nostril with the left thumb. The fingers are stretched up yet relaxed. Inhale long and deep through the right nostril and focus all your attention on the breath. Finally, inhale and exhale deeply and relax. Length: 3-5 minutes
Helps you to have a clear mind.

2 In the kneeling pose, stretch the arms straight up, press the palms together and practice sat kriya for three minutes. Inhale deeply, hold the inhale, and engage mula bandha. Imagine that your energy is streaming out from the navel point to the entire body. Exhale, relax, and then repeat this breath exercise for three minutes. Inhale, engage mula bandha, and guide all your energy with your mind from your navel to your fingertips. Exhale, release the pose, and relax.
Allows access to all the energy stored in the navel point.

3 In the simple seated pose, grasp the ankles and begin the camel ride. Let SAT vibrate in your mind with each inhale, and let NAM vibrate in your mind with each exhale. Finally, exhale, straighten the spine, and hold the breath briefly. On the exhale, release the pose and relax. Repetitions: 108
Leads the freed Kundalini energy along the spine and supports its flexibility.

4 Squat and spread the legs so that the heels are together and the knees point outward. Support yourself between your legs with spread fingers. Raise up onto your toes, engage the throat lock, and make sure that your spine is straight. On the inhale, stretch out your legs and bring your forehead toward your knees. On the exhale, return to the starting position and make sure that the head remains an extension of the spine. Repeat the cycle. On the last repetition, inhale deeply in the extended position, hold the inhale briefly, and release the pose on the exhale. Repetitions: 26
Strengthens the entire sexual system and activates its natural energy flow.

5 In the kneeling pose, lay the palms softly on the thighs and hold the spine straight. Inhale and turn the head to the left; exhale and turn it to the right. On each inhale, think SAT, and on each exhale, think NAM. Finally, turn the head forward again. Inhale and exhale deeply and relax. Length: 3 minutes
Helps the energy of the throat chakra flow, activates blood flow to the head, and stimulates the thyroid gland.

6 Come into the simple seated pose. Grasp the shoulders with the thumbs behind and the fingers in front. Make sure that the elbows are at shoulder height. Bend the upper torso to the left on the inhale and to the right on the exhale. Your breath is long and deep. Finally, inhale, straighten your torso, exhale, and relax. Length: 3 minutes
Increases flexibility of the spine, distributes energy in your entire body and balances the aura.

7 In the simple seated pose, engage mula bandha. Concentrate on the third eye and pay attention to your breath. Think SAT on the inhale and NAM on the exhale. Length: at least 6 minutes
Leads to a deep, self-healing meditation.

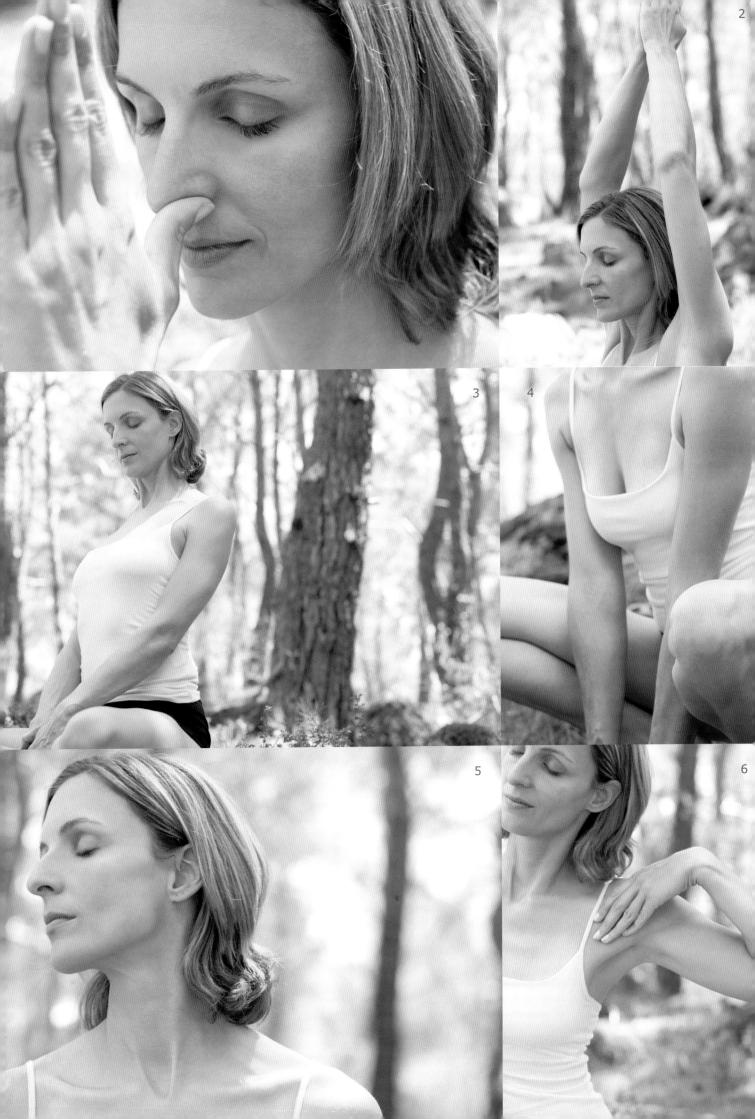

GIVE YOUR LIVER STRENGTH

1 Lie on your left side and support your head with your left hand. Bend the right knee, grasp the right big toe with your index and middle fingers, and stretch the leg straight up. The left leg remains extended on the floor. Begin the breath of fire. Length: 4 minutes

2 Lift yourself into wheel pose from a supine position. First inhale and then exhale through the nose. Then inhale and exhale through the mouth. Repeat this switch from mouth to nose with each breath. Length: 4 minutes

3 Repeat exercise 1. Breathe the breath of fire, but this time, do so the mouth. Length: 2 minutes

4a Stand upright with the feet somewhat wider than shoulders' width apart. Bend your upper body down. Stretch your arms through your legs as far as possible and place your hands on the floor. Hold this position. Length: 1 minute

4b Remain in this position, roll the tongue, and stick it out slightly. Begin the breath of fire through the tongue. Length: 3 minutes

5 Repeat exercise 1. Inhale through the nose and exhale powerfully and explosively through the open mouth. Length: 30 seconds

6 In the simple seated pose, stretch the arms out horizontally to the side. Come to a standing position on the inhale and let yourself sink back to the simple seated pose on the exhale. Complete this exercise without using your hands to help. Repetitions: 52

7 Stand upright with feet shoulders' width apart. Put your hands on your hips and begin to rotate your upper body, keeping it straight. Length: 2 minutes

8 Relax deeply in the simple seated pose.

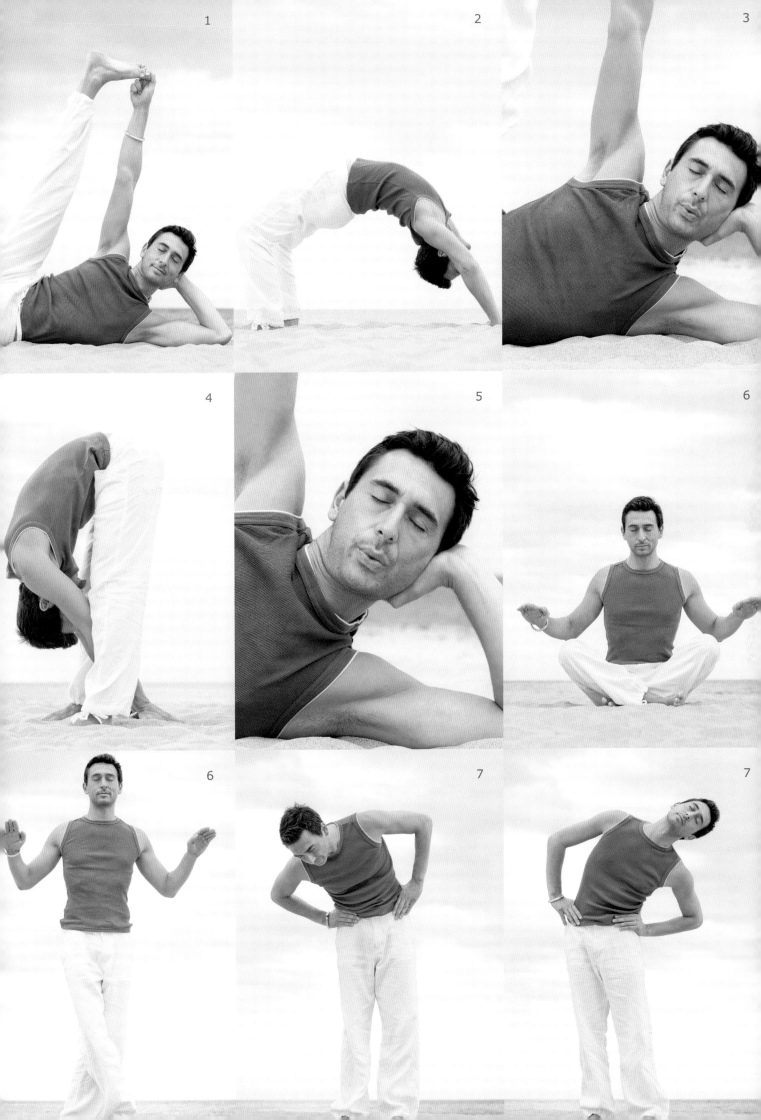

NABHI KRIYA

1 Lie on your back and stretch out your legs. On the inhale lift the left leg straight up, and lower it again on the exhale. Repeat with the right leg. Breathe powerfully and deeply and repeat the raising and lowering of the leg alternately with each breath. Length: 10 minutes
This exercise activates the lower digestive organs.

2 On the inhale, lift both legs straight up together. Knees and heels are touching. Lower them back to the starting position on the exhale. The arms are stretched up during the entire exercise, with the palms facing each other. Length: 5 minutes
Stimulates the upper digestive organs and the solar plexus.

3 Bend the legs, bring the knees to the chest, and embrace them. The head lies on the floor. Relax with long, deep breath. Length: 5 minutes

4 Embrace the legs as in exercise 3. From this position, stretch the legs up and out so that they create a 60° angle with the floor. At the same time, stretch the arms out to the sides with the palms facing upward. Exhale and embrace the legs again. Repeat the cycle. Length: 15 minutes
Exercises 3 and 4 recharge the electromagnetic field and activate the navel center.

5 Lie on your back and stretch both legs out. Bring the right knee to the chest and grasp it with the hands. Inhale and lift the extended left leg straight up as fast as possible. Lower it to the floor on the exhale. Continue this motion. Switch sides halfway through the time and repeat. Length: 2 minutes

6 Repeat exercise 5. Length: 2 minutes
Exercises 5 and 6 stabilize the hips and spine.

7 Stand and lift your arms straight up with palms facing up. On the exhale, bend forward until your hands touch the floor and engage mula bandha. On the inhale, stand up straight and then repeat the motion. Breathe long and deeply. Length: 2 minutes

8 Repeat exercise 7 with increased speed. Length: 1 minute
Exercises 7 and 8 invigorate the spine and strengthen the aura.

9 Relax with long deep breath or meditate. Length 10-15 minutes

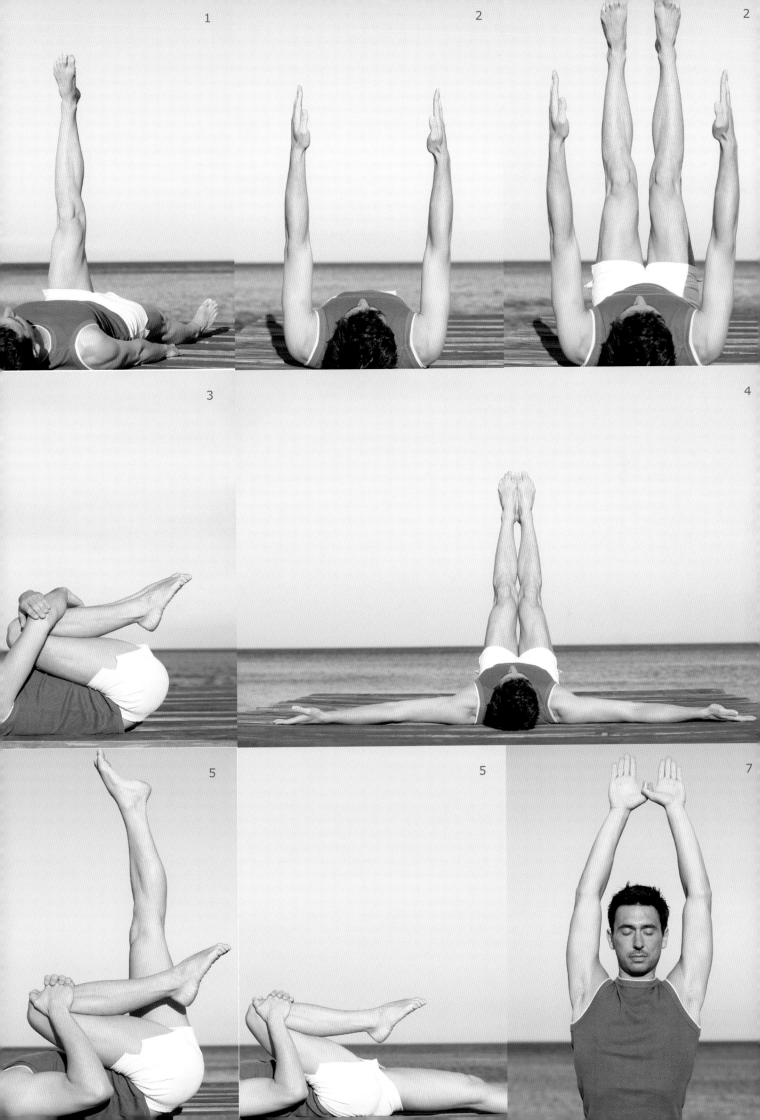

KRIYA FOR PURIFICATION OF THE SELF

1 Squat with feet flat on the floor. Stretch one leg back as far as possible and lay the top of the foot on the floor. Shift your weight to the front foot, so that the back leg is unburdened. Bend forward slightly with a straight back, bring the hands into prayer, and concentrate on the third eye. Inhale deeply and hold your breath for seven to eight seconds. Exhale. Complete this breath cycle a total of four times. Switch legs and repeat.

2 In the simple seated pose, brace your hands on your hips. Lift the shoulders as high as possible toward the ears and lift the diaphragm. Inhale and exhale very deeply in this position. Length: 2-3 minutes
Helps the energy in the lungs flow and stimulates the thyroid gland.

3 Hook your hands together in front of your chest in the bear grip with your arms parallel to the floor and the right palm facing downward. Inhale deeply. Exhale powerfully and completely. Hold the exhale as you engage mula bandha. Hold the next inhale, engage mula bandha and, in your mind, make the prana energy rise from the bottom of your spinal column. Length: 3 minutes
Strengthens the heart and opens the heart chakra.

4 In the simple seated pose, stretch the arms straight out to the side and bend the hands up so that the palms face outward. Roll your eyes up and concentrate on the third eye. Inhale and hold while you engage mula bandha strongly for twenty seconds. Repeat the cycle with the next inhale. Length: up to 3 minutes

5 In the simple seated pose, press the palms together firmly in front of the chest. The fingers point upward. Length: 2 minutes
Exercises 4 and 5 support healing of the hands and activate circulation.

6 Relax deeply.

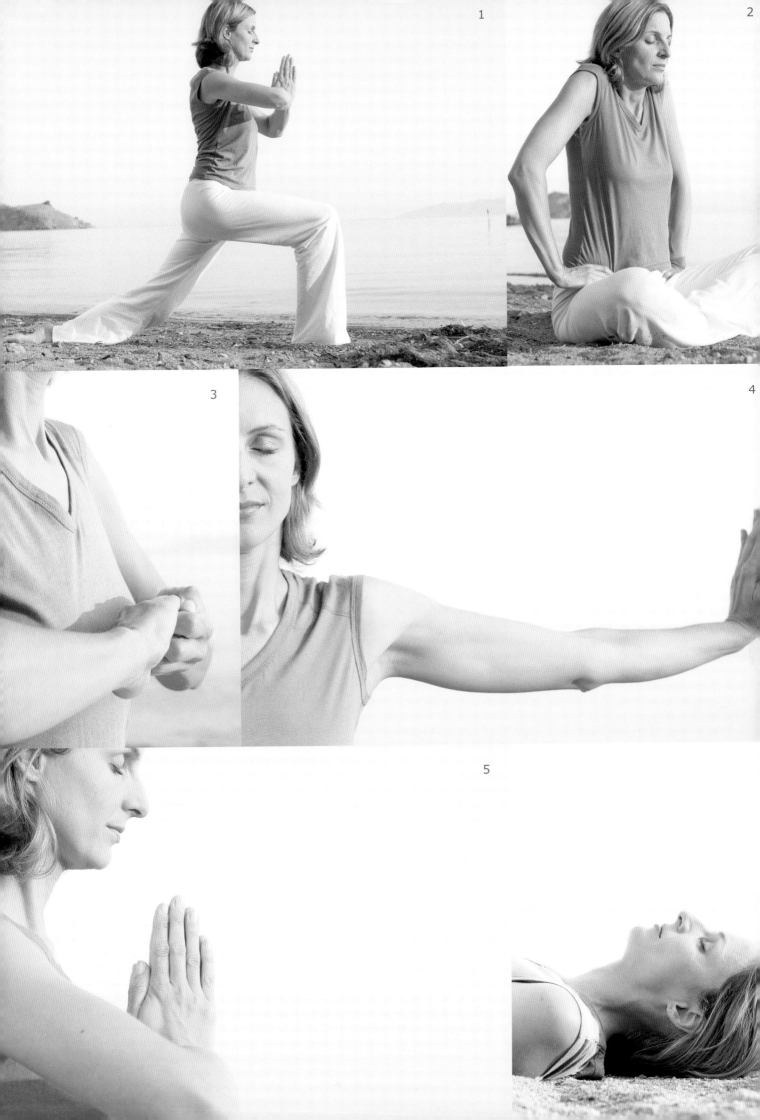

1

2

3

4

5

KRIYA FOR PELVIC BALANCE

1 Sit on the floor with bent legs, place your feet on the floor, and support yourself back on your arms. Lift the pelvis to come into bridge pose. Make sure that the calves and arms are perpendicular to the floor. The knees, pelvis, and shoulders create a line parallel to the floor. Let the head hang back, engage mula bandha, and breathe long and deeply in this position. Length 1-3 mintues
Strengthens the back and supports aerobic metabolism.

2 Lift yourself into the wheel pose and begin the breath of fire. Length: 1-3 minutes
Strengthens the lower back, lightens the energy flow, and supports aerobic metabolism.

3 Lie on your stomach with your legs together. Brace your knee against the floor. Interlace the fingers behind your back in the Venus lock. Lift the extended arms and legs from the floor as far as possible and begin the breath of fire. Finally, inhale and exhale deeply and relax. Length: 1-3 minutes
Supports digestion and strengthens the stomach muscles.

4 Stand with your legs spread widely, stretch your arms straight up, and place the palms together. Inhale, bend your upper body to your left leg with a straight back, and touch your left foot with your fingertips. Stand up on the inhale and bend to the other side on the exhale. Repeat the cycle with deep, powerful breath. Length: 1-3 minutes
Balances the movement of the pelvis and coordinates the supporting muscle groups.

5 Sit in Kundalini lotus and begin the breath of fire. Finally, inhale and exhale deeply and relax. Length: 1-3 minutes
Channel the sexual energy and helps potency.

6 Come to your hands and knees and begin cat-cow. On the inhale, lift the head up and back while stretching the right leg as far up as possible. Make sure that the knee is extended. On the exhale, bring your chin and knee toward your chest simultaneously so that, ideally, they touch. Repeat this motion with powerful breath for 1-3 minutes. Inhale and exhale deeply, switch legs, and repeat for 1-3 minutes. Finally, inhale and exhale deeply, release the pose, and relax.
Strengthens the abdominal and back musculature and helps to maintain sexual potency.

7 Relax.

It is advised that you do a warm-up exercise before this fairly strenuous exercise sequence, so that the spine is warm and flexible. Beginners should take care to practice this exercise slowly and carefully.

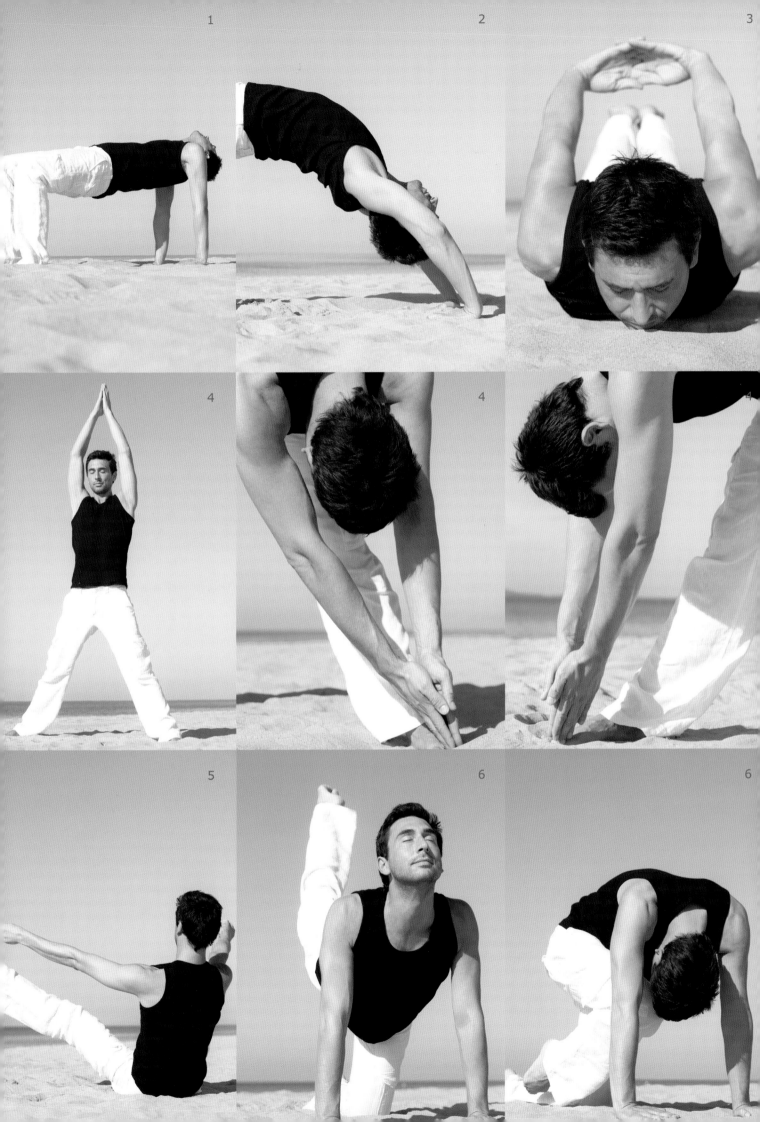

COORDINATING BODY, MIND, AND SOUL

1 In the simple seated pose, massage the tragus in front of the ear canal with your thumbs. Length: 1 minute

2 In the simple seated pose, interlace the fingers in the Venus lock and lift the arms straight over the head. Stretch upward by slowly making spirals with your torso and arms, starting at the base of the spine. Feel how you sit straighter and straighter. Make sure that the arms remain extended for the entire exercise. Length: 4 minutes
Stretches the spine at least ½-1 inch.

3 Stay in the same position and spiral up three more times. Bend forward until your forehead touches the ground; the arms remain stretched above the head. Sit up and repeat the forward bend. Length: 3 minutes

4 Lie on your back with your arms next to your body. Lift your arms, legs, and upper body so that only the seat still touches the floor. Hold your balance and direct your attention to your toes. Move the navel in and out with your breath, but do not go as far as the breath of fire. Length: 5 minutes

5 Repeat exercise 2. Repetitions: 52 spirals

6 In the simple seated pose, stretch the arms above the head. Shake your hands out vigorously, so that your entire body moves along with them. Length: 1 minute
Removes the effects of toxins in the body.

7 Squat and spread your legs so that the heels touch and the knees point outward. Support yourself on your hands between your legs. Come up on the tips of your toes, engage the throat lock, and make sure that your spine is straight. Inhale, stretch out the legs, lift the seat, and lower the forehead toward the knees. Return to the starting position on the exhale and lift the head so that it remains an extension of the spine. Repeat the cycle. On the last repetition, inhale deeply in the position with your legs extended, briefly hold the inhale, and release the pose on the exhale. Repetitions: 52

8 In the kneeling pose, stretch the arms over the head and interlace your fingers in the Venus lock. In this position, bend forward until your forehead touches the floor. Sit up and repeat the exercise. Move to the rhythm of Jaap Sahib, a Sikh prayer from Northern India. Repetitions: 108

9 In the simple seated pose, lay the hands one on top of the other on the chest. Continue to hear Jaap Sahib. Length: 13 minutes

10 Remain in the simple seated pose with hands crossed on the chest. From your deepest heart, sing the last lines of Jaap Sahib:
> Chattr Chakkr Warti
> Chattr Chakkr Bhugate
> Suyambhav Subhand Serbe Da Serbe Jugte
> Dukaalang Pranassi De-alang Serupi
> Sadaa Ange Sange Abhangang Bibuthe

Length: 6 minutes
This mantra banishes fears.

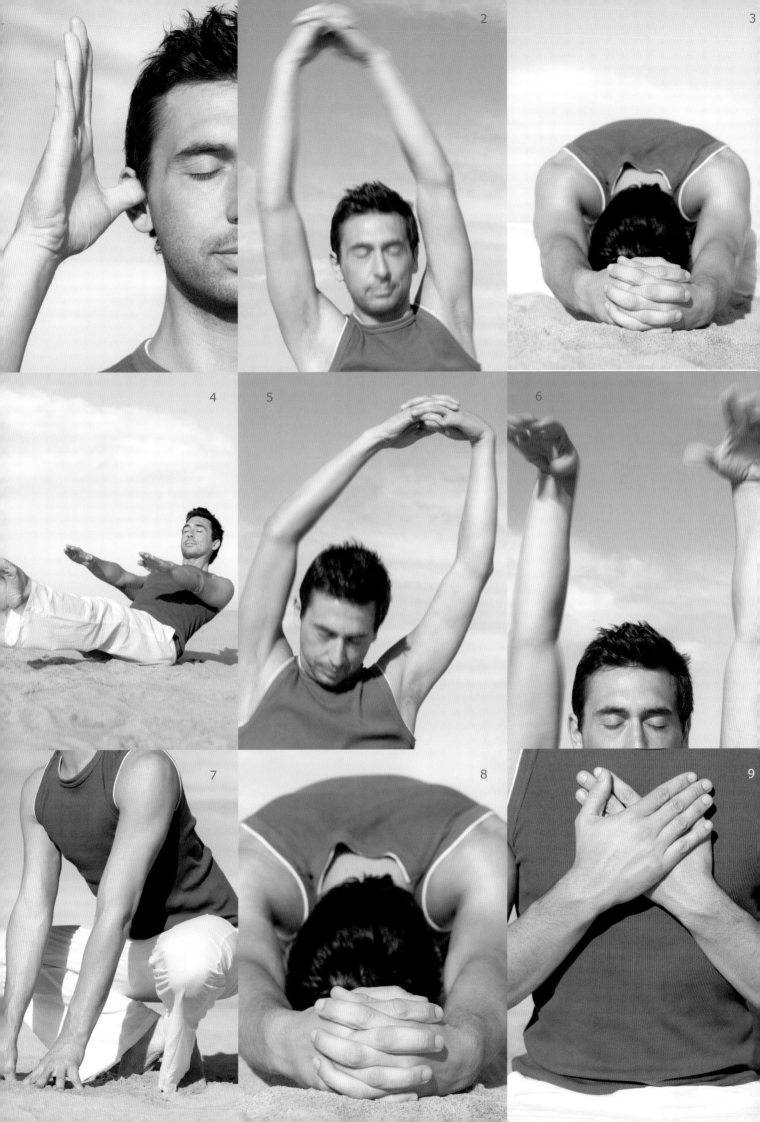

MEDITATION AND SELF-RELIANCE

1a Sit upright and extend the legs. Stretch the arms straight out ahead of you with the palms facing downward. Inhale and lean back with a straight spine until it creates a 60° angle with the floor. Lift the extended legs up as far as possible. Hold the inhale in this position as long as you can. Exhale and lower the legs.

1b Bend your straight upper body forward, grasp the toes and pull them toward you. Remain in this position and breathe naturally. Length: 11 minutes

2 Take a few strong breaths in the same position. Inhale, sit up, and repeat exercise 1a. Repetitions: 3-4
Exercises 1 and 2 align the aura balance. Through pressure on the liver, cleansing processes are activated. Increases courage to face life.

3 In the kneeling pose, lay the hands on the thighs and begin the camel ride. Powerfully whisper SAT when you bend the spine forward and NAM when you bend it back. The sound of your breath should be similar to the hiss of a snake. Finally, inhale and exhale deeply four times. Length: 8 minutes
Opens the heart center and activates love and compassion.

4 In the simple seated pose, put the hands together in front of the chest and cross the thumbs. Press the hands together as firmly as possible. Through doing this, pressure will be exerted on the center of the chest. Concentrate on the tip of the nose and meditate. Length: 10 minutes
This exercise stimulates the liver.

5 Remain in the simple seated pose, stretch the arms straight out to the sides. Move your body to the left side on the inhale and to the right side on the exhale. The arms remain parallel to the floor for the entire exercise. Length: 3 minutes
This exercise stimulates sexual energy.

6 In the simple seated pose, grasp the ankles and begin a quick camel pose. Emphasize the forward movement so that the sex organs experience gentle pressure. Length: 3 minutes

7 Lie on your back and relax.

8 In the simple seated pose, bring your hands into ghyan mudra. Concentrate on the tip of your nose, turn your head to the right and chant SAT NAM. Turn your head to the left and sing WAHE GURU. Continue in an equal rhythm. Length: 11 minutes
This exercise can be practiced for up to thirty-one minutes.

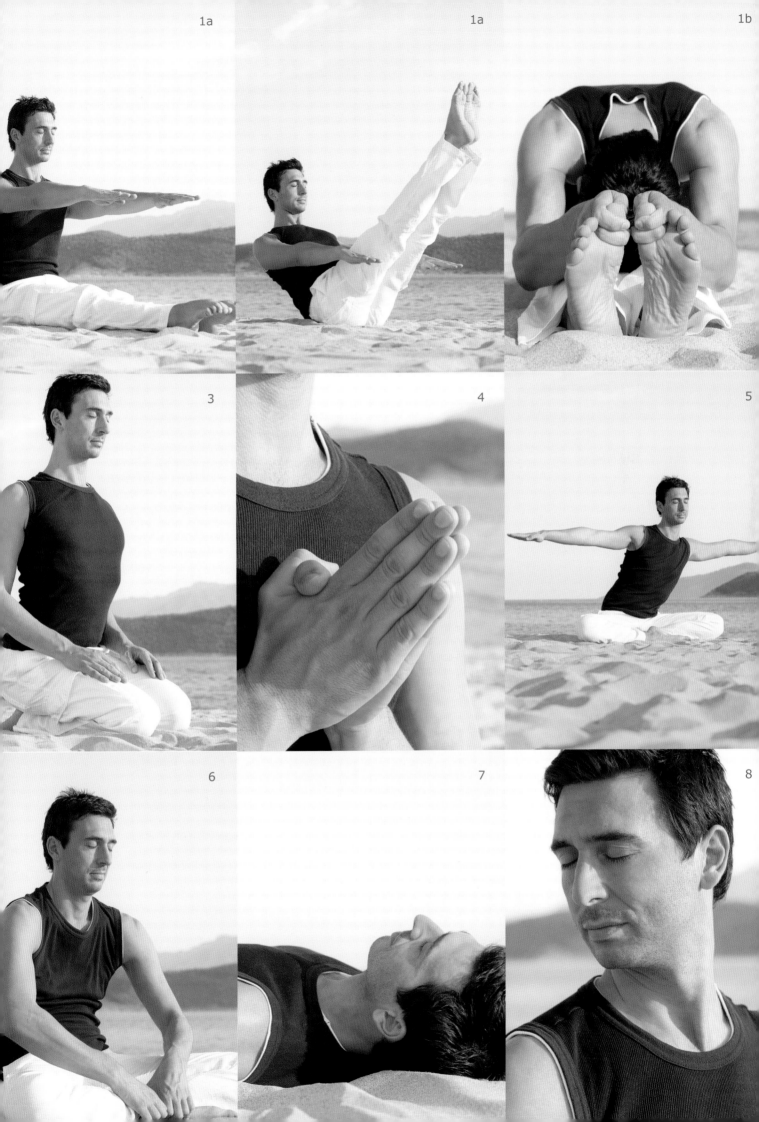

1a

1a

1b

3

4

5

6

7

8

NOBILITY

Nobility is a virtue that affects every soul
As innocence affects every Heart
Woman has one virtue: to be noble till death
Living nobly is very blessed
Living your truth is happiness

Nobility is a virtue in the presence of God
The greatest virtue that can be expressed
Nobility through everyone whatever they may be
Before the one God equality

A noble woman gives birth to a noble life
Noble children and surroundings be
A noble woman lives nobly and looks noble
Even if she lives in poverty

Unlike a mirror, distorted when it is cracked
Noble habits are a noble life
Don't barter character values for benefits
A noble person does not forget the presence of god

Nobility is manufactured inside
Training to exert self-esteem
To see herself confirms her virtuous face
Selfless living grace through time and space

EFFECTS ACCORDING TO YOGI BHAJAN

106 Sat Kriya:
There is a multitude of effects of sat kriya. The sacral chakra is strengthened and its natural energy flow is activated. Sexual impulses can be better channeled and transformed into creative and healing processes in the body.
This kriya helps in particular with serious imbalances or mental problems, because these are always connected to an imbalance of the energies of the three lower chakras.
The pumping motion of the navel point massages the internal organs gently and strengthens the heart. The Kundalini energy is stimulated and channeled. (Sadhana Handbook)

108 Varuyas Kriya:
Varuyas kriya makes the body sweat; the cheeks begin to burn slightly. The exercise activates the pituitary gland, regulates rising sexual energies, and strengthens resistance and the nervous system. It brings the aura back into balance. (Sadhana Handbook)

110 Wake-Up Series:
Yogi Bhajan did not comment on the effects of this kriya. (Relax and Renew*)

112 Activating the Kundalini Energy:
This powerful kriya is a wonderful preparation for a deep meditation. With the help of this kriya, women and men can work on raising sexual energy and will feel orgasms through their entire spines during intercourse. (Relax and Renew*)

114 Basic Spinal Energy Series:
With this series, the spine is systematically activated from the base to the neck. All twenty-six vertebra

are stimulated and the chakras receive an energy surge. This is why this kriya is very useful as a preparation for meditation.

With regular practice, the circulation of spinal fluid is strengthened and thus greater mental clarity and strength are achieved. (Sadhana Handbook)

116 Kriya for Strengthening Disease Resistance:
Yogi Bhajan did not comment on the effects of this kriya. (Keeping up with Kundalini Yoga)

118 Kriya for Overcoming Insomnia:
This kriya helps with insomnia and should be practiced for ninety days, either in the morning after waking or in the evening before sleeping. (Sadhana Handbook)

120 Exercise Series for the Kidneys:
Yogi Bhajan did not comment on the effects of this kriya. (The Aquarian Teacher)

122 New Opportunities and Green Energy:
"The more I open, the more I draw in. I must not fight against it. I have the opportunity to attract new chances and new paths. . . . This set opens the heart center and in this way opens new paths and possibilities and enables success and prosperity. . . . Begin to understand that new paths and outcomes can come to you in different forms. Begin to understand that you have earned it. Begin to understand that you are in holy love." Y. B. (Relax and Renew*)

126 Cleansing Series for Beginners:
This series makes the body more beautiful and gives it a sense of light. (Sadhana Handbook)

128 Surya Kriya:
Surya kriya activates the sun breath, which provides power, expressiveness, enthusiasm, and inner warmth. Weight is regulated and digestion is activated. The mind is cleansed and analytical thoughts and activity orientation are supported. It stimulates positive, creative energy and the Kundalini energy itself. (Sadhana Handbook)

130 Give Your Liver Strength:
"If you cannot make a conscious connection to the body, your mind will not be able to build a connection to you. Whoever practices this set will be armed for life." Y. B. (Owner's Manual for the Human Body)

132 Nabhi Kriya:
Nabhi kriya brings the digestive system quickly under control. (Handbook for Teachers and Students)

134 Kriya for Purification of the Self:
This kriya cleanses and energizes body and mind. If this series is practiced before a relaxing or healing massage, it will protect from fatigue and help to concentrate the energy.

136 Kriya for Pelvic Balance:
If the pelvis and its supporting muscle groups are out of balance, physical stress symptoms can appear, such as fatigue, low endurance, and pain in the lumbar spine. This kriya helps to guard against these grievances. With regular practice, it will help with balance, increase energy, and preserve potency. (Keeping up with Kundalini Yoga)

138 Coordinating Body, Mind, and Soul:
Yogi Bhajan did not comment on the effects of this kriya. (Self Knowledge)

140 Meditation and Self-reliance:
This series supports self-reliance and energizes on all physical and mental levels. (Handbook for Teachers and Students)

*The guide to this kriya is taken from Gururattan Kaur Khalsas's *Relax and Renew* and thus could not be verified for authenticity and accuracy by the Kundalini Research Institute.

"Meditation is a duty to the self. In the moment in which you become aware of your own self, you become beautiful. Because, in the moment in which you concentrate on the self, your frequency changes and the universe around you changes in the exact same way. That is a funny law." —Y. B.

MEDITATION
MEDITATIO = PONDERING, DIRECTED INWARDS

Meditation is a vital element of KUNDALINI YOGA. The goal of meditation is to open and to come to know the mind through attentiveness and concentration.

The first stage of meditation is concentration. Through concentration we try to collect any thoughts and feelings, focus on a point, and to calm ourselves. In KUNDALINI YOGA, the most common concentration points are the crown of the head, the third eye, the tip of the nose, the chin, or the navel point. Complete mastery of concentration is the basis for meditation.

"A trait that all types of meditation have in common, even at the procedural level, gives us a clue to the attitude we are trying to describe: all meditation is a dwelling upon something. . . . Meditation is concerned with the development of a presence, a modality of being, which may be expressed or developed in whatever situation the individual may be involved. This presence or mode of being transforms whatever it touches. If its medium is movement, it will turn into dance; if stillness, into living sculpture; if thinking, into the higher reaches of intuition; if sensing, into a merging with the miracle of being; if feeling, into love; if singing, into sacred utterance; if speaking, into prayer or poetry; if doing the things of ordinary life, into ritual in the name of God or a celebration of existence. . . . While practice in most activities implies the development of habits and the establishment of conditioning, the practice of meditation can be better understood as quite the opposite: a persistent effort to detect and become free from all con-ditioning, compulsive functioning of mind and body, habitual emotional responses that may contaminate the utterly simple situation required by the participant. This is why it may be said that the attitude of the meditator is both his path and his goal." (Naranjo & Ornstein)

SEVEN WAVE SAT NAM MEDITATION

Sit upright and place the hands together in prayer. Close your eyes and fix your attention on your third eye. Inhale deeply and on the exhale, sing SAT NAM for seven beats. SAT has six beats, NAM only one. Let the tone of SAT flow through the first six chakras in six waves, beginning with the root chakra. Make sure that you always concentrate on the particular chakra that the wave is flowing through. On the seventh and last beat, let the energy and sound of NAM beam through the crown chakra into the aura. On the next inhale, begin again. Length: 15 minutes

This meditation is a good introduction to KUNDALINI YOGA. It opens the mind for new experiences. Those with experience can use this meditation in preparation of others, to relax, and to come to peace.

"To change yourself means also to change behavior patterns. By vibrating the sound of SAT NAM in this way, you activate the energy of the mind that eliminates and creates habits." —Y. B.

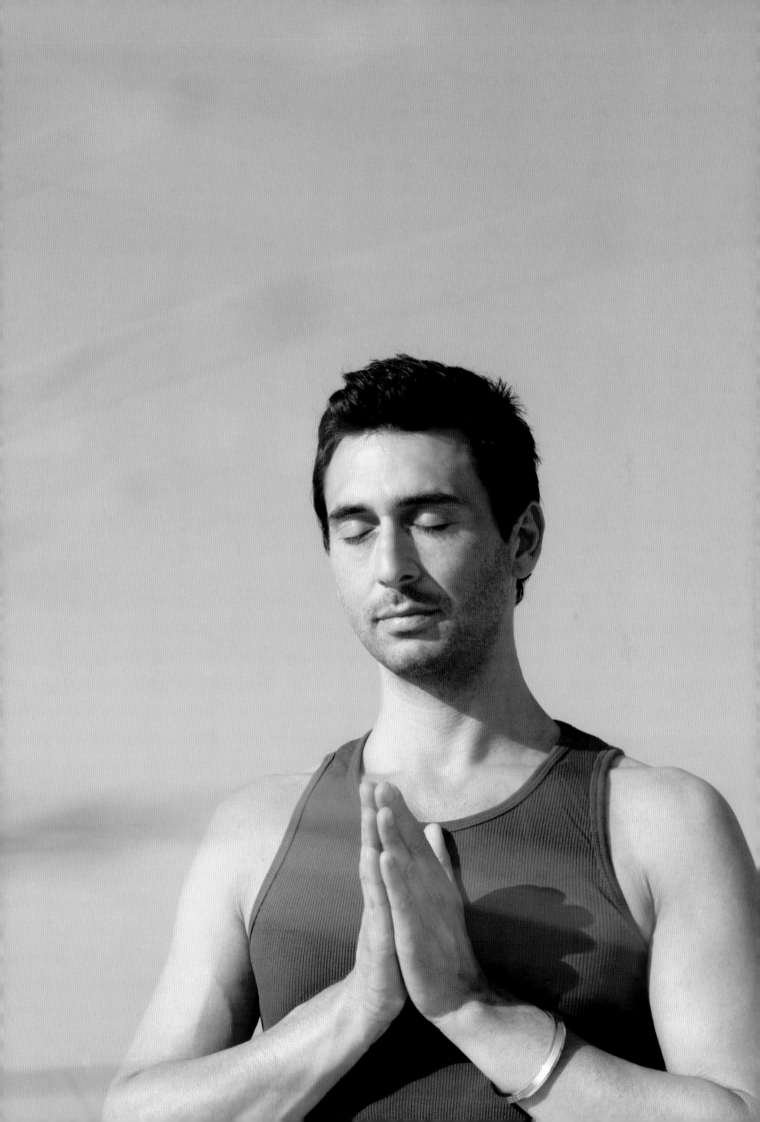

EMOTIONAL BALANCE

Drink a glass of water before beginning this meditation. Come into the simple seated pose and close your eyes. Cross your arms in front of your chest and place your hands in your armpits. The palms face the ribcage. Lift your shoulders to your ears and engage the throat lock. Make sure that you do not cramp your neck muscles. Hold this position and let the breath become peaceful all by itself. Length: 3-11 minutes

To work against strong agitation, turbulence, and imbalance, it is important to drink a lot of water and to reduce the breath from fifteen to four breaths in a minute.

"During mental or emotional imbalance, full attention should be given to hydration and breath count." —Y. B.

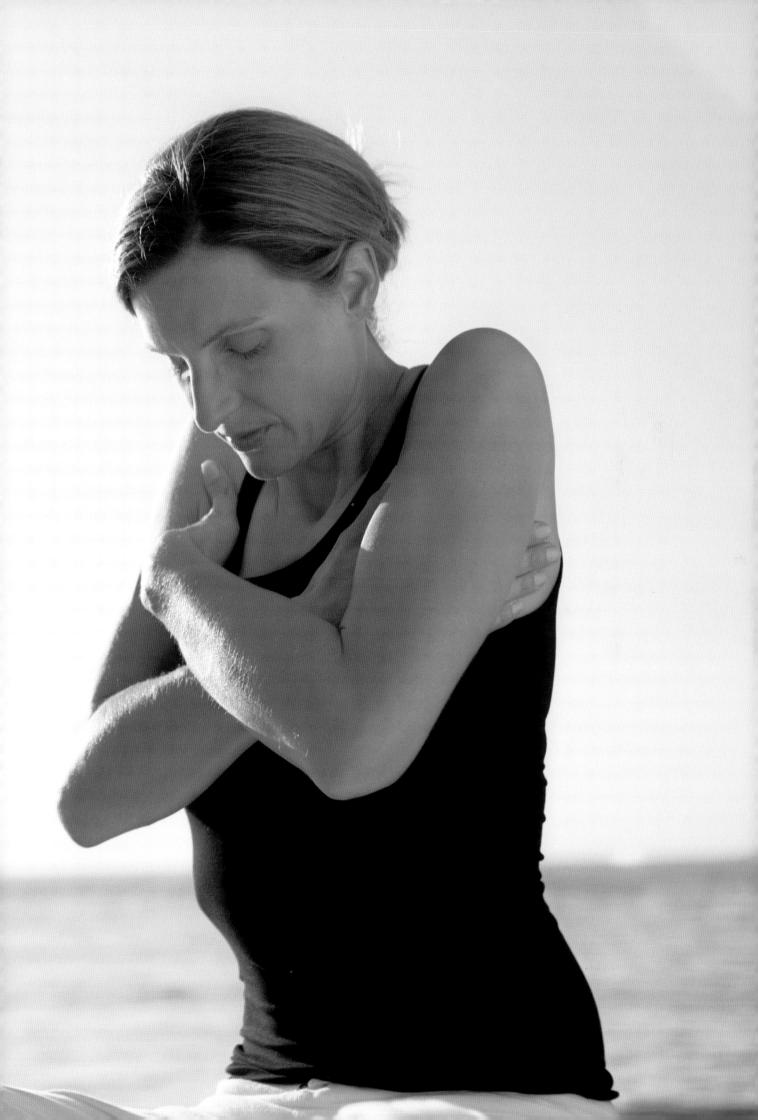

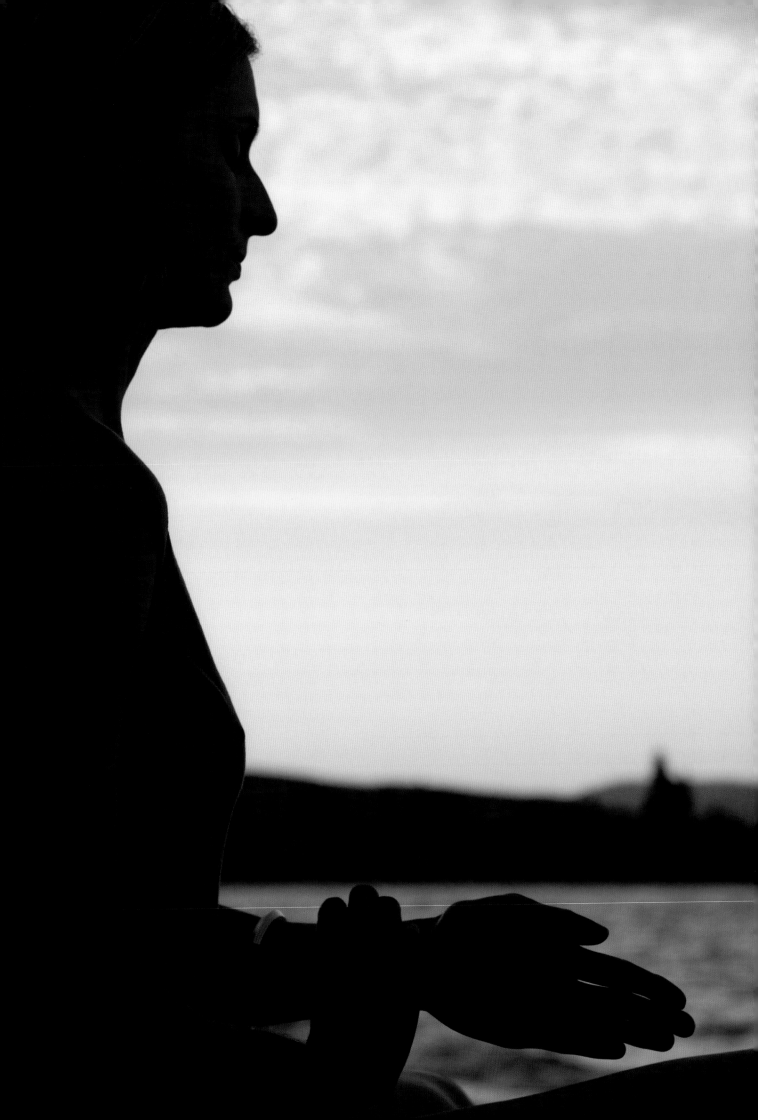

CONCENTRATION IN ACTION – LEARNING MEDITATION

Sit upright in the simple seated pose and feel the pulse of your left wrist with your right hand. The fingertips should create a line so that you can feel your pulse in each finger. Close your eyes softly and concentrate on the third eye. With each heartbeat, feel the mantra SAT NAM. Length: 11-31 minutes

This meditation is particularly suited to beginners. It teaches the ability to concentrate on something and to bring a muddled, scattered mind to peace.

MEDITATION TO FREE YOURSELF FROM DEPRESSION & FOR THE CAPACITY TO COPE WITH LIFE

In the simple seated pose, stretch the arms out straight in front of you. Make your right hand a fist and grasp it with the left hand. The heels of the hands touch. The thumbs are together and point straight up. Gaze toward your thumbs, close your eyes almost all the way, and look through the small gap between the thumbs. Make sure that your back is straight.

Inhale for five seconds and then exhale completely for five seconds. Hold the breath for fifteen seconds after the exhale and then inhale again. Begin with a meditation time of three to five minutes. With increasing practice you can gradually increase the time, but do not exceed eleven minutes. If you have enough experience, you can increase the pause between the exhale and the next inhale up to one minute. Length: 3-11 minutes

This meditation allows you to build a direct relationship to the pranic body and grants you the power to master your own life.

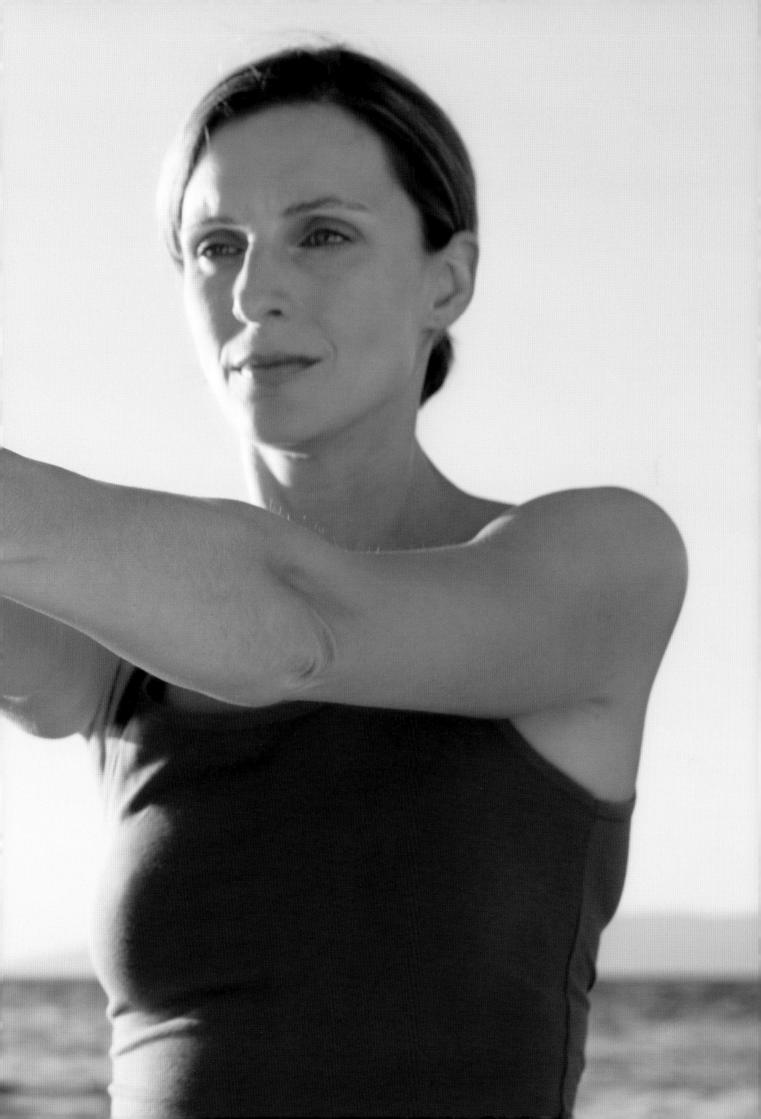

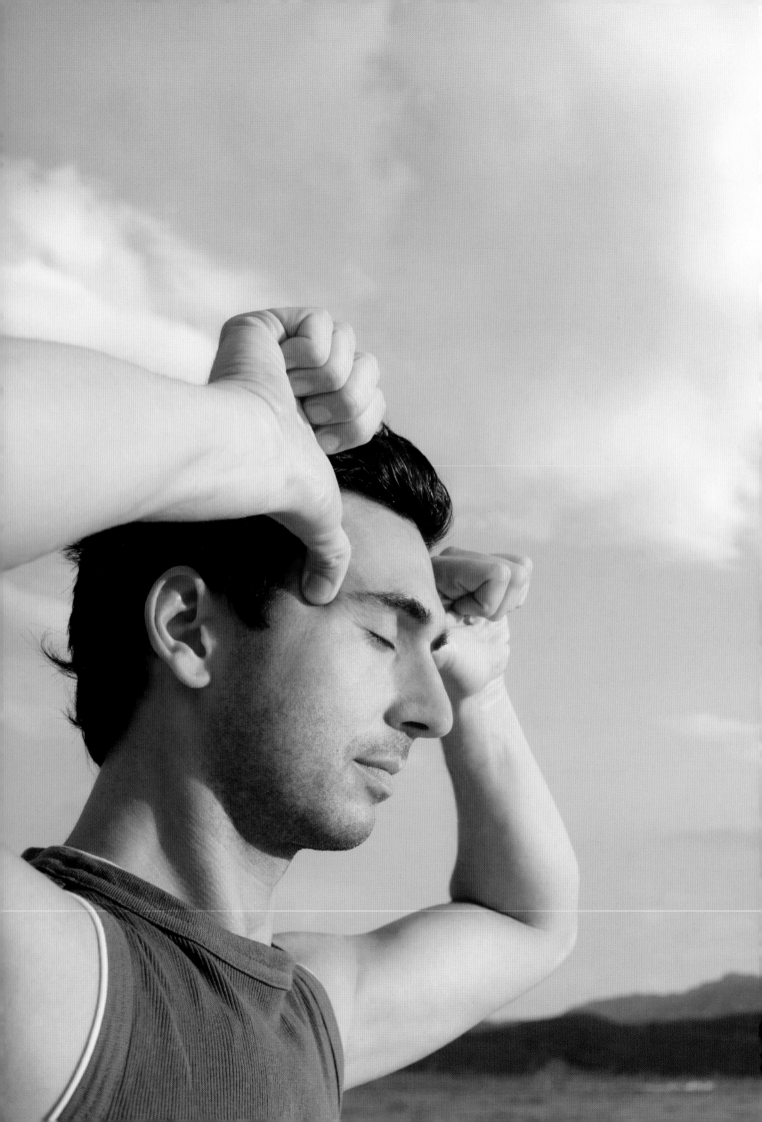

MEDIATION AGAINST ADDICTIVE HABITS

Sit upright in the simple seated pose and push the lower six vertebra forward. Make your hands into fists and press your extended thumbs against your temples. Press your molars together in a constant rhythm so that you can feel the resulting movement with your thumbs. At the same time, concentrate on your third eye and sing SA TA NA MA in your mind. Feel the mantra at your temples. Length: 3-31 minutes

According to Y. B., this meditation evokes change processes in the brain and in this way helps to dissolve addictions to nicotine, caffeine, sugar, and alcohol.

KIRTAN KRIYA

Come into the simple seated pose and lay your hands on your knees with palms facing downward. Concentrate on the third eye and begin to chant the mantra SA TA NA MA, with each cycle lasting three to four seconds. With each syllable, press the thumb against the corresponding finger:

SA   Index finger
TA   Middle finger
NA   Ring finger
MA   Little finger

Sing for two minutes at a normal volume, two more minutes at a whisper, and then sing four more minutes soundlessly. Then, sing at a whisper for two more minutes and again at normal volume for two minutes. To finish, stretch the arms up, straighten your spine, take a deep breath, and relax.

The ratio of the times for loud-quiet-silent-quiet-loud should always be 1-1-2-1-1. Stick to the times you have chosen within one meditation session. If you want to practice the meditation over several days or weeks, you can raise the times gradually to 5-5-10-5-5 minutes. The three volumes of loud, quiet, and silent correspond to the three languages of the consciousness. Loud stands for the human consciousness, the worldly, the material. Quiet represents the living and the wish for belonging. Silent symbolizes the godly, the infinite.

"To practice this meditation leads in the individual psyche to complete mental balance. Each time you close the thumb and finger into a mudra, the effect lingers in your consciousness and the electric charge in your body changes.

The balance of the electromagnetic fields that flow around our bodies also manifests in the fingertips. In contrast to the other fingers, the thumb and index finger are electrically negative.(...) Meditation is science and art at the same time. It is an art in the way that it forms the consciousness and refines sensation and cognitive faculty. It is a science because the outcome is always the same. Each and every action has a particular effect on the psyche. That is why it is important to practice meditation exactly." —Y. B.

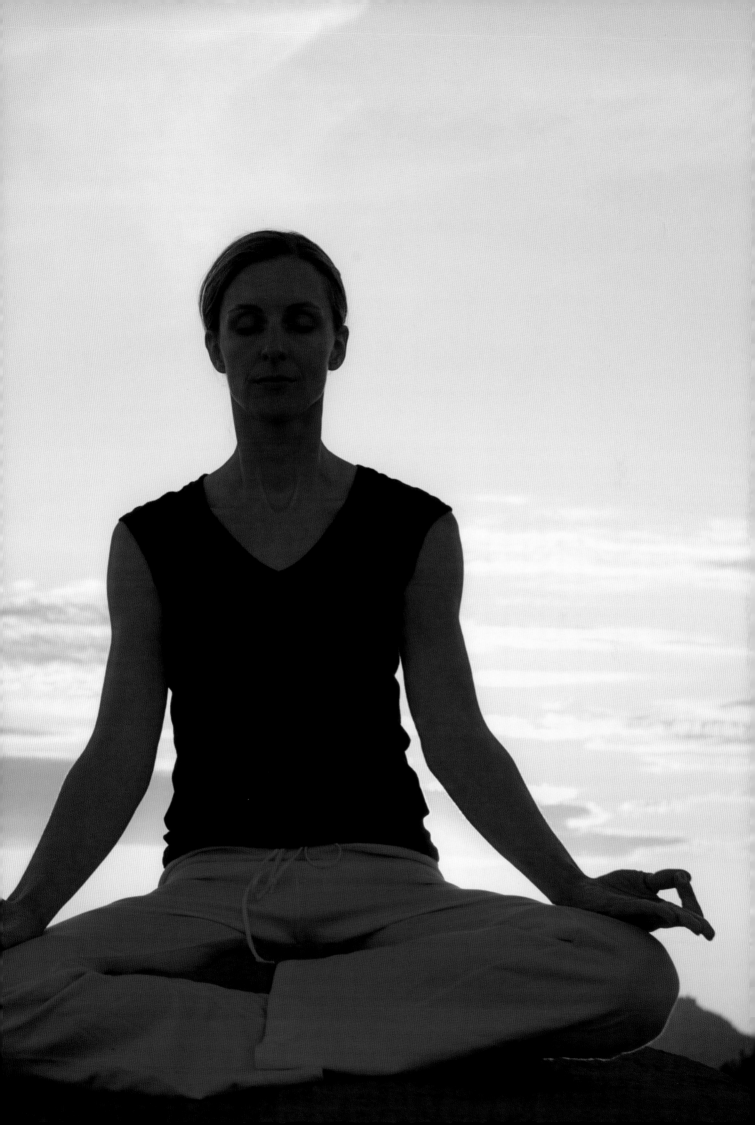

BEGGAR'S MEDITATION

Come into the simple seated pose. Lay the right hand across the left and form a bowl in front of your heart chakra. Concentrate and gaze into this bowl. Begin to inhale deeply and slowly through the nose and exhale deeply and slowly through the mouth. Purse your lips as though you wanted to spit air into the bowl. Direct your attention through the whole meditation on a desire, no matter how lowly it may seem to you. On the inhale, meditate on this desire and blow it into the bowl on the exhale. Length: 11-31 minutes

Too many desires block the personality, according to Y. B. With the help of this meditation, these blocks can be dispersed in appropriate parts of the brain and the underlying mental patterns are transformed.

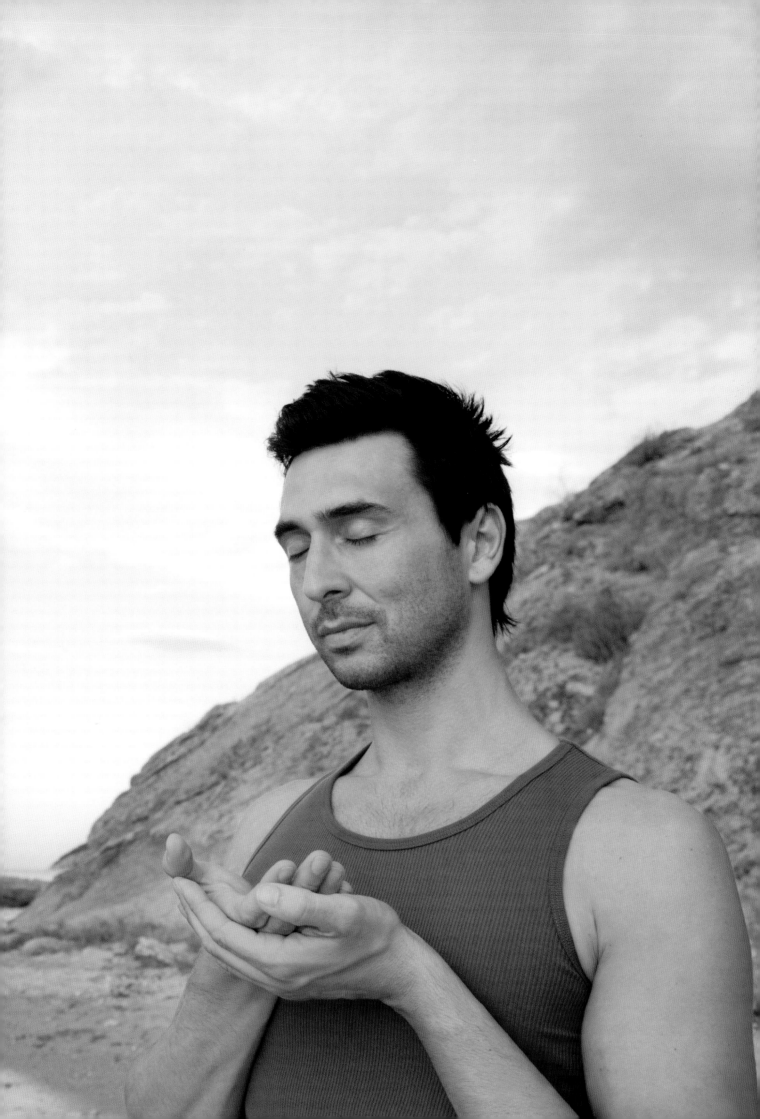

SMILING BUDDHA KRIYA

In the simple seated pose, bend your little fingers and ring fingers and press them against the palms with your thumbs. Index and middle fingers remain extended. Angle your forearms so they create a 30° angle to your upper arms. The upper arms are parallel to each other and the palms face forward. Make sure that your sternum is lifted. Concentrate on your third eye. In your mind, chant SA TA NA MA. Finally, inhale and exhale deeply, open and close the hands several times, and relax. Length: 11 minutes

When there is an outstanding, lovely person who moves your heart and who you admire, then according to Y. B. you should practice this meditation to reach the same state of consciousness as this person. This hand position, which you have surely seen on icons or figures, is a gesture of bliss, which causes the energy of the heart center to flow.

This meditation helps you to be completely yourself as you create beauty and peace in your surroundings.

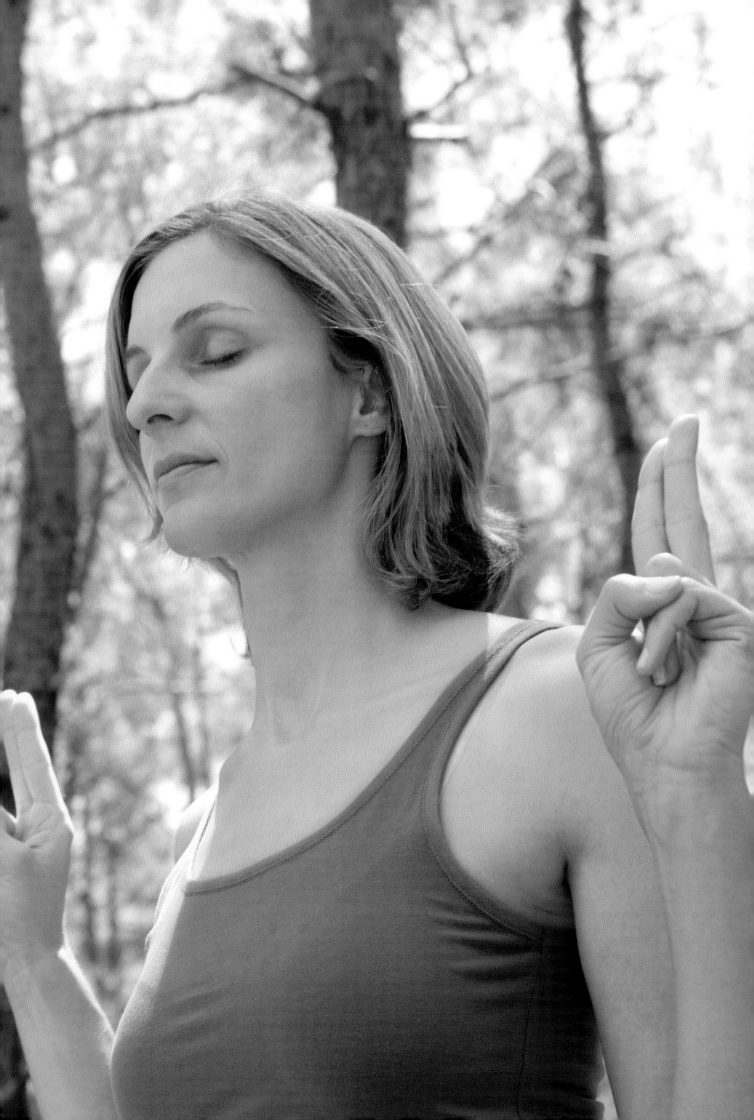

UNGALI PRANAYAMA

In the simple seated pose, lay the hands relaxed in ghyan mudra on the knees. Make sure that your back is straight. Inhale and exhale deeply several times and, after the last complete exhale, begin with the particular breath of this exercise. Inhale in fifteen equal parts and exhale in fifteen equal parts. In your mind, chant SA TA NA MA while

inhaling in fifteen parts while chanting SA fifteen times in your mind,
exhaling in fifteen parts while chanting TA fifteen times in your mind,
inhaling in fifteen parts while chanting NA fifteen times in your mind,
exhaling in fifteen parts while chanting MA fifteen times in your mind.

A complete SA TA NA MA cycle lasts about thirty seconds. Length: begin with 3 minutes and lengthen the time 1 minute daily (up to 31 minutes)

Be aware of the intensity of this meditation and do not overtax yourself.
Have a glass of water ready to that you can drink something if you become dizzy during the meditation.

"Ungali pranayama affects the central nervous system. . . . It coordinates its duties and activates the functions of the left and right halves of the brain. . . . This sound, which is created in your mind, is meant to be a part of your inner, extremely capable, self-guided self.
Ask your inner self if it likes the mantra and how it reacts to it. These sounds and rhythms speak the language of your self." —Y. B.

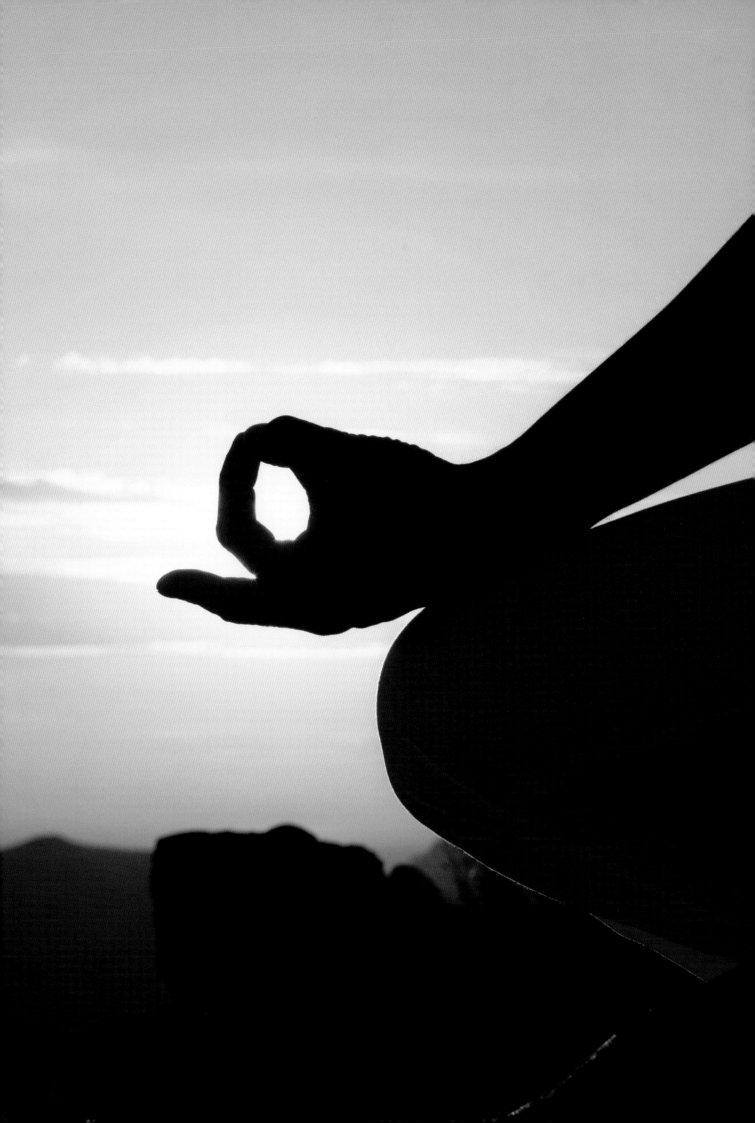

HEALING

The following healing meditation is practiced in a group. The healing people sit in a circle and send healing energy to the person who lies relaxed and with closed eyes in the middle.

As healers, come into the simple seated pose in a circle around the people to wish to be healed. Rub your hands to start the energy flowing. Stretch your arms forward so that they create a 30° angle to the floor. The hands are also stretched and the palms face downward. Sing the mantra RA MA DA SA SA SE SO HANG. Let this mantra vibrate up along the spine, one syllable through each chakra. The last syllable leaves the body vibrating powerfully at the crown.

Finally, inhale deeply, hold your breath and send healing energy to the people in the middle of the circle. Exhale and inhale again, stretch the arms straight up, meditate silently for a moment, and exhale. Inhale again, send healing energy to the others in the circle and to all life on earth, and then exhale.

Feel a bright, golden light in your heart and notice how it spreads to each and every cell in your body. Connect it with the light of the group and feel how it first heals the entire room, then your neighborhood, the whole city, and the whole country. Let the whole earth be bathed in your healing light. Feel how your entire environment is healed and the hearts of all people are filled with love and peace. Fly over the earth and send it your golden, beaming energy. Unite with the light of the universe. Come back slowly and know that you contain this light and can share its healing power with others.

Repeat this cycle until all participants in the middle have received healing energy.
Length: 3-31 minutes

This meditation can also be practiced alone, either for yourself or to heal a fellow person.

Sit upright in the simple seated pose. Lay the upper arms tight against the ribcage and bend the forearms up so that they create a 60° angle to the floor and point out at 45°. The palms face upward. Close your eyes, inhale deeply, and chant RA MA DA SA SA SE SO HANG.
Length: 11 minutes

An eleven-minute daily practice is enough to create enormous healing power in your hands, which can be used for yourself and others.

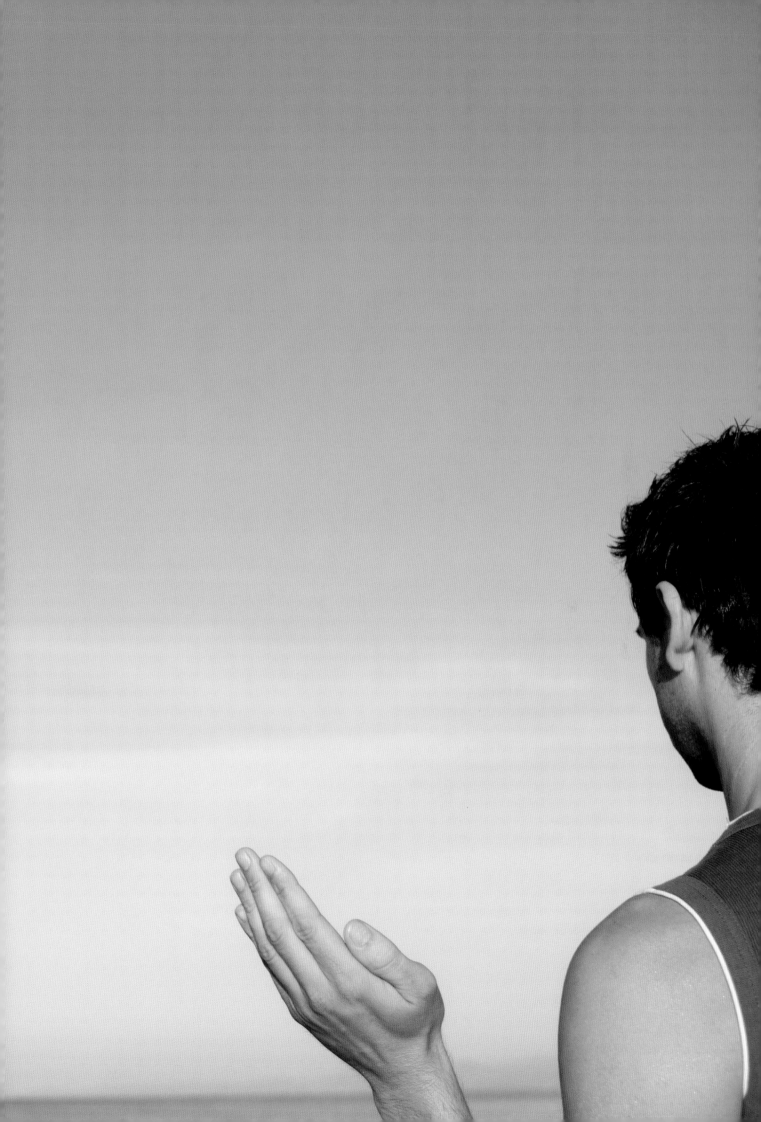

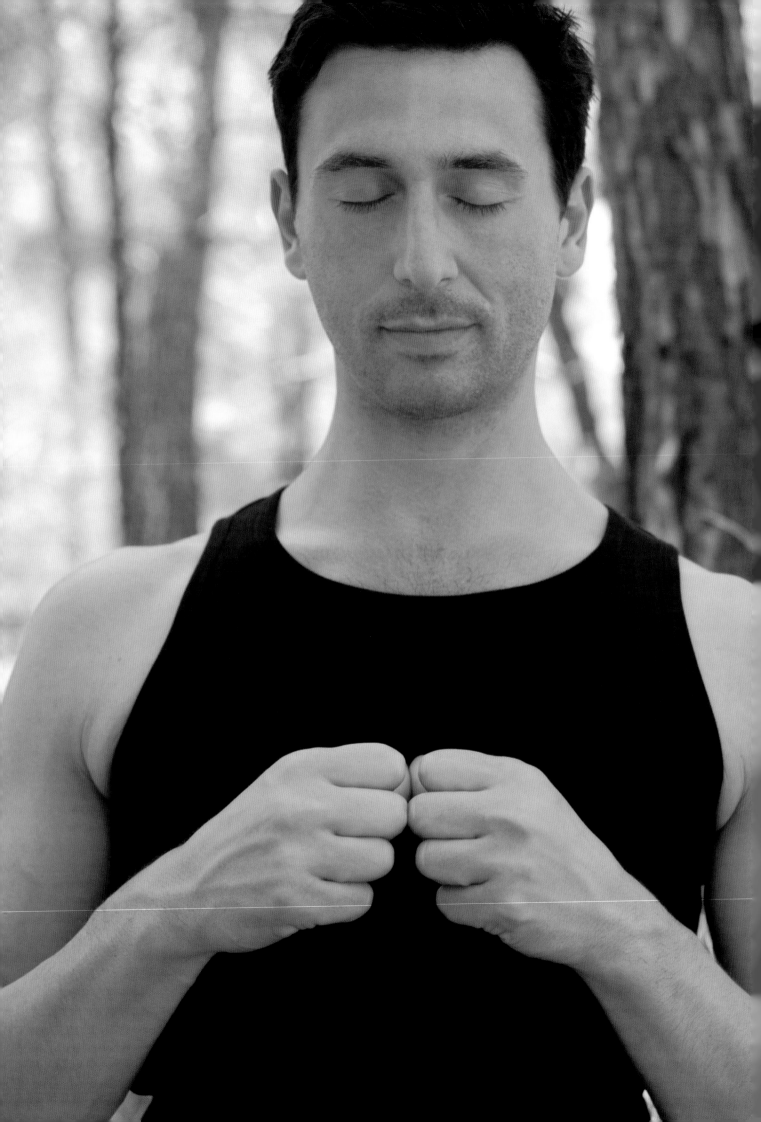

MEDITATION FOR CHANGE

Lift the chest slightly while in the simple seated pose. Bend your fingers and touch the heels of your hands with your fingertips. Bring the hands together in front of the chest, so that only the knuckles of the middle fingers and the bases of the thumbs touch. The thumbs are extended toward the chest and pressed together gently.

Hold the hands in this mudra and breathe long and deep for thirty-one minutes. Concentrate on the flow of breath and feel the energy between your thumbs and knuckles.

Finally, inhale and exhale deeply and relax for five minutes. Length: 36 minutes

If it is possible for you to practice the meditation for thirty-one minutes and remain sure and relaxed, you can practice an additional thirty-one minutes after relaxing.

"Change is the law of the universe. Everything changes. Whatever may change, one thing seems to always stay the same: the attachment to your ego. . . . To become happy in all the changes and to let your soul fully shine, you should be ready to give up your self for the Higher Self." —Y. B.

MEDITATION FOR SELF-ASSESSMENT

For this meditation you need another person, a teacher, to whom you listen attentively and whom you repeat. In this meditation, contemplate with full awareness to what extent your mind is behind what you say and what seems untrue to you.

Sit up straight and close your eyes. Repeat the following words after your teacher:

I am unique.
Very graceful.
Completely pious.
Absolutely perfect.
Flawlessly beautiful.
Beyond words.
I am completely virtuous.
A living truth.
In conversation with friends.
In conversation with enemies.
In my political life.
In my social life.
In my material life.
In my personal life.
In my private life.
I am absolutely correct.
Righteous.
Wise.
And completely good.
I understand.
Everything.
My knowledge is absolutely complete.
I created God.
He did not create me.
I am not joking, it is the truth.
I am talking about it.
Therefore I am the creator.
I can create the word "God."
By writing it on the wall.
By pronouncing it with my tongue.
By communicating with humans.
I created the radio.
The television.
I print the newspaper.
I broadcast everything that I can.
I am master and proprietor of the entire universe.

Open your eyes and check the extent to which you agree with what you said. Finally, sing the mantra ONG loudly and powerfully for three to eleven minutes.
In a group meditation the women and men should begin to sing at different times, as in a round.

"No energy is more powerful than that of the spoken word. Because we are not aware of the effect of what we say, we say what comes to mind and act upon what we feel in the moment. Thus a duality arises between action and word. . . . This meditation allows you to assess how well you can coordinate your actions and speech. If you cannot, you will experience a conflict as you initiate the duality in your personality. Constantly assess yourself, until the mind only says what is really true." —Y. B.

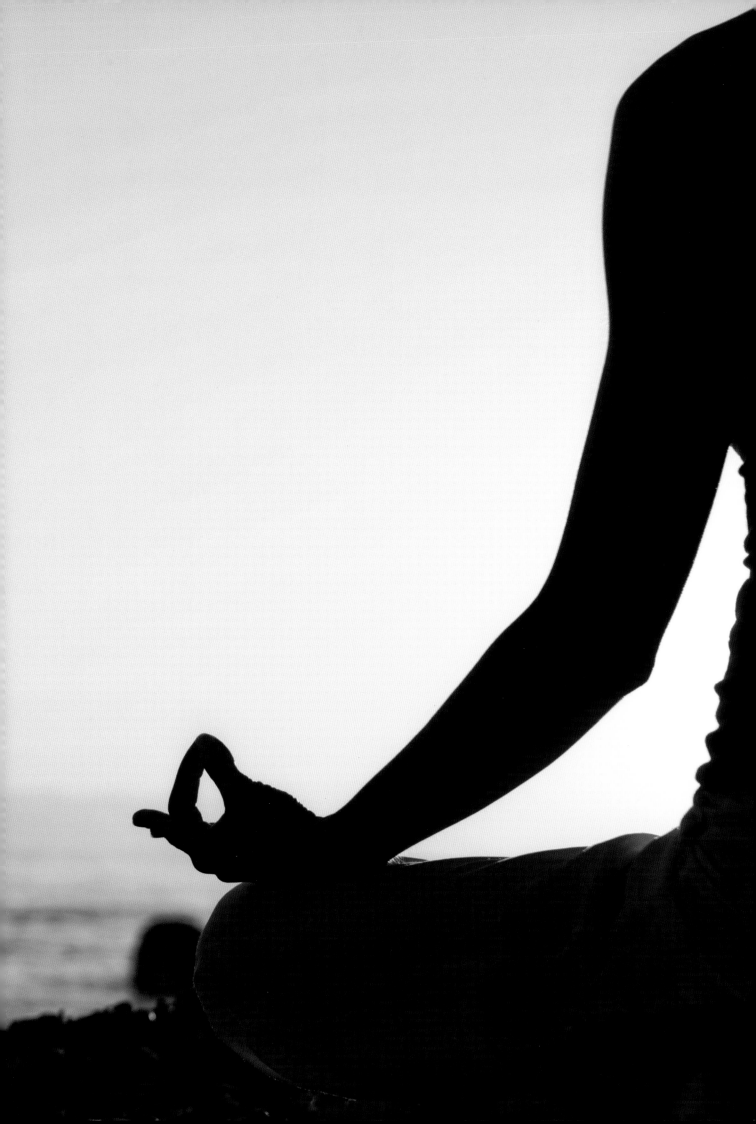

"The strength of a person does not lie in what he possesses. The strength of a person lies only in that which he is able to give. Only those who have the capacity to reach out into the universe can give something. When the universe is not a part of your mind, your heart is not able to give." —Y. B.

MANTRA
MAN = MIND
TRA = PROJECTION, GIVING DIRECTION

Mantras are syllables, words, or short sentences that are recited and serve to relax the mind and cleanse the subconscious. They are an acoustic means to guiding concentration and they serve as a tool for entering a raised state of consciousness.

A mantra is chanted before, during, or after an exercise or meditation, either loudly, quietly, or in your mind (silent). Chanting means reciting the mantra repeatedly in a sort of spoken song. The vibrations created by a mantra stimulate particular energy points in the palate. This stimulation has a calming effect on the organs, the brain, and the psyche. It furthers your ability to concentrate and centers the mind.

KUNDALINI YOGA works with many mantras that work on different levels. There are mantras which activate the heart center and others which strengthen the nervous system or improve communication. Most of the mantras that appear in KUNDALINI YOGA originate from Gurmukhi, the holy language of the Sikhs from Northern India.

Before each KUNDALINI YOGA exercise session, you should sing a mantra three times to prepare yourself, open up, and build a connection with your Higher Self. The three repetitions align with our three levels of being: bodily, mental, and spiritual.
Sit in the simple seated pose and bring your hands together in prayer. Take several deep breaths, inhale and sing three times:

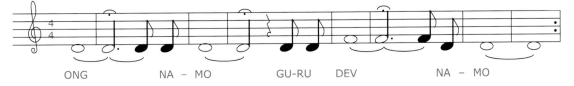

ONG   NA – MO   GU-RU DEV   NA – MO

To end the session, a song and a mantra are sung to return to a grounded state in the outer world. Come into the simple seated pose again, bring the hands into prayer and sing

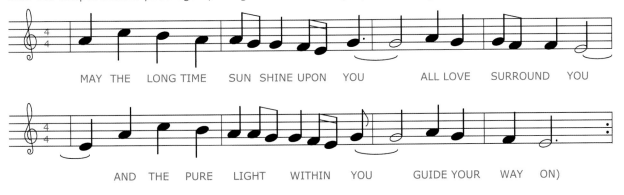

MAY THE   LONG TIME   SUN SHINE UPON   YOU   ALL LOVE   SURROUND   YOU

AND   THE   PURE   LIGHT   WITHIN   YOU   GUIDE YOUR   WAY   ON)

Finally, inhale deeply and sing three times:

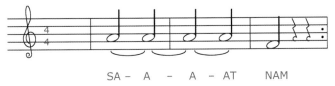

SA – A – A – AT   NAM

Adi Mantra ONG NAMO

I bow before subtle godly wisdom ONG NAMO
Before the internal godly teacher GURU DEV NAMO

Mangala Charan Mantra   AAD GURAY NAMEH

I bow before the original truth   AAD GURAY NAMEH
I bow before wisdom   JUGAAD GURAY NAMEH
Which is true over all eras   SAT GURAY NAMEH
I bow before true wisdom   SIRI GURU DAYVAY NAMEH
I bow before the great, unseen wisdom

Guru Gaitri Mantra	GOBINDE MUKANDE
Sustaining	GOBINDE
Freeing	MUKANDE
Enlightening	UDARE
Infinite	APAARE
Destroying	HARIANG
Creating	KARIANG
Nameless	NIRNAME
Free from want	AKAME

Siri Gaitri Mantra/Siri Mantra	RA MA DA SA
Sun	RAA
Moon	MAA
Earth	DAA
Impersonal Infinity	SAA
You	SAY
Entirety of Infinity	SAA SAY
Personal feeling for fusion and identity	SO
Infinity, vibrating and real	HANG
"I am you"	SOHANG

Gurmantra WAHE GURU

I am in ecstasy WHA – HE GURUU
When I experience indescribable wisdom

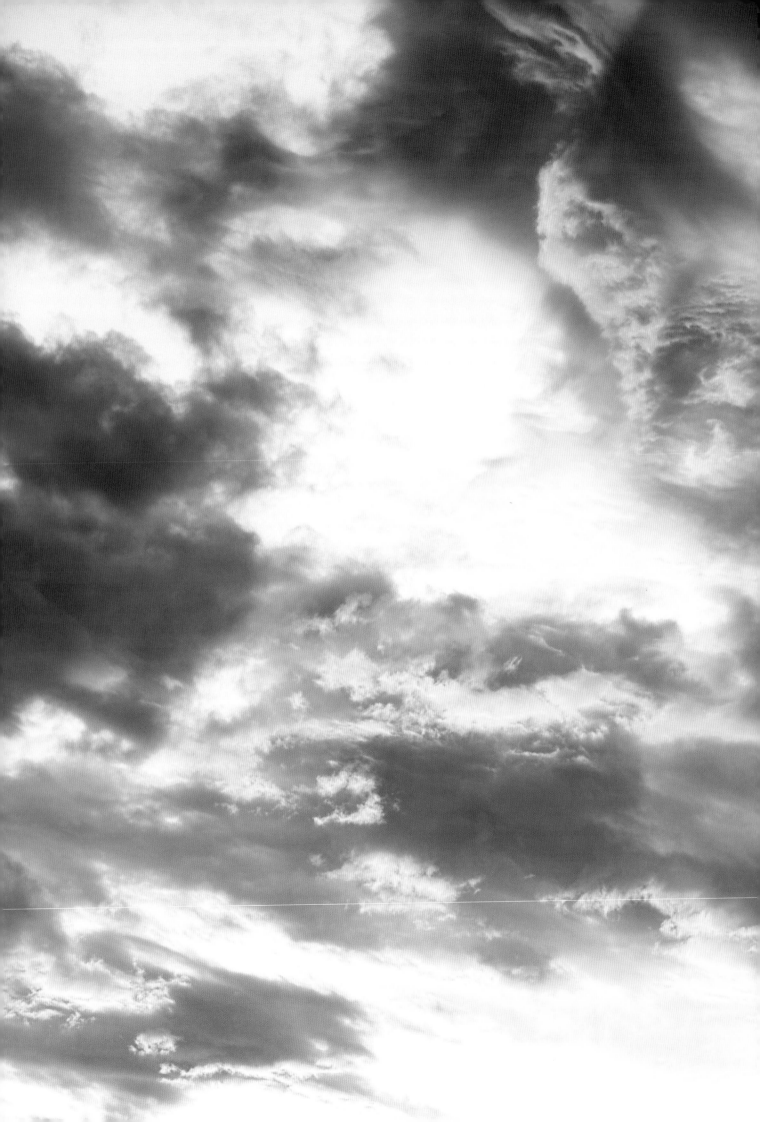

Adi Shakti Mantra **EK ONG KAR SAT NAM**
SIRI WAHE GURU

Creator and Creation are one **EK ONG KAAR**
That is our true identity **SAT NAAM**
The ecstasy of this wisdom is awesome beyond all words **SIRI WAHE GURU**

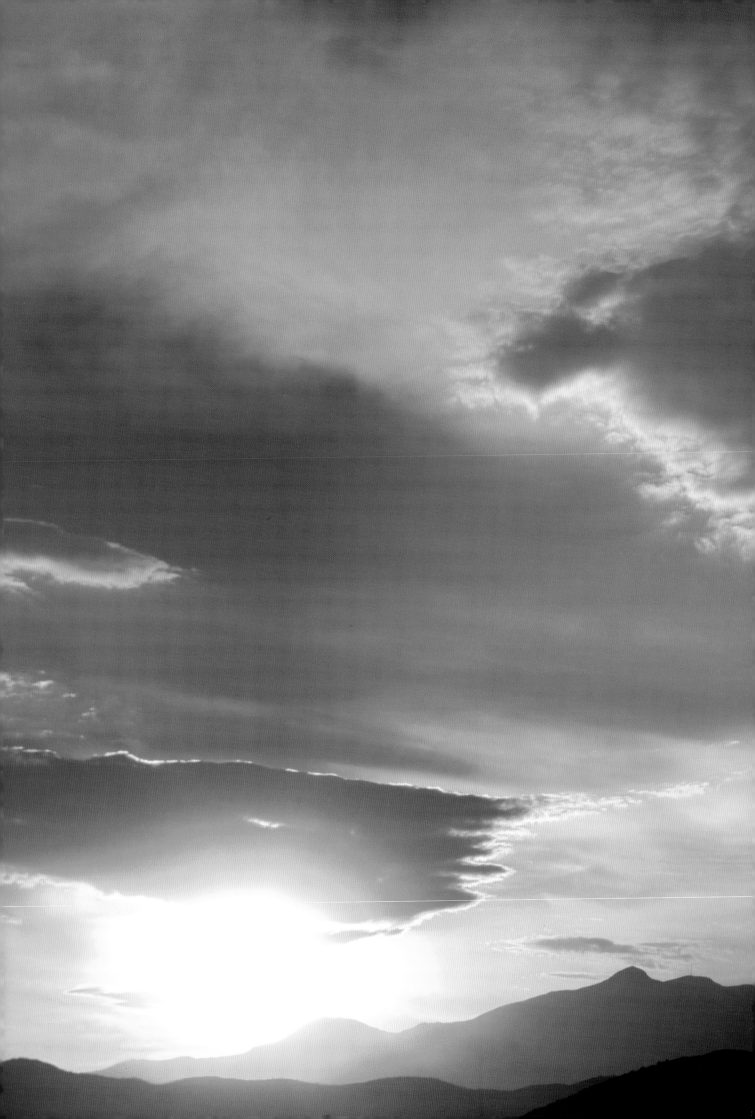

Mul Mantra	EK ONG KAR
Creator and Creation are one	EK ONG KAR
That is our true identity	SAT NAM
He who does everything	KARTA PUREK
Beyond fear	NIRBHAO
Beyond revenge	NIRVAIR
Image of infinity	AKAL MURET
Unborn	AJUNI
Self-enlightened	SAIBHANG
Complete in yourself	GURPRASAD
That is the gift of the guru	
Meditate	JAP
Original truth	AAD SUCH
True through all time	JUGAD SUCH
True in this moment	HEBHI SUCH
Oh Nanak, always true	NANAK(E) HOSI BEE SUCH

Kundalini Shakti Mantra   AAD SUCH

True at the beginning   AAD SUCH
True through all time   JUGAD SUCH
True in this moment   HEBHI SUCH
Nanak says, this truth will always be   NANAK HOSI BEE SUCH

Kundalini Bhakti Mantra ADI SHAKTI

I bow ADI SHAKTI
Before the original power ADI SHAKTI
ADI SHAKTI
NAMO NAMO

I bow SERBE SHAKTI
Before the all-encompassing power and energy SERBE SHAKTI
SERBE SHAKTI
NAMO NAMO

I bow PRITHAM BAGAWATI
Before that which god created PRITHAM BAGAWATI
PRITHAM BAGAWATI
NAMO NAMO

I bow KUNDALINI MATA SHAKTI
Before the creative power of Kundalini MATA SHAKTI
The power of the godly mother NAMO NAMO

Mantra of Ecstasy   WAHE GURU WAHE JIO

Awesome beyond all description   WA – HE GURU WA – HE GURU
Is the infinite wisdom   WA – HE GURU WA – JIO

Bij Mantra SAT NAM

Truth is our identity SAT NAAM
We resonate in our existence

GLOSSARY

A

Adi Mantra (Adi = original)
   The first mantra used to prepare before a yoga session.

Apana
   Elimination energy; a part of prana.

Asana
   Third level of eight-limbed yoga: body pose.

Ashtanga
   Yoga composed of eight levels built on each other; also called Raya Yoga Kriya.

Aura
   Electromagnetic field that surrounds people.

Ayurveda (= the knowledge of life)
   The healing practice of yoga.

B

Bhakti Yoga (= the way of devotion)

   One of the four classical yoga paths, with the goal of attaining unity with God through prayer and love.

Bandha (= lock, seal)
   Locking technique for the body locks to optimize the flow of prana in the nadis.

Bear Grip
   Hand position in which the hands are hooked together in front of the chest.

Bhagavadgita
   The most important Hindu text; describes the essence of yoga in a cohesive text form.

Breath of Fire
   The basic yoga breath method. Energizing, cleansing, quick belly breaths through the nose.

Buddhi Mudra
   Seal of communication; hand position in which the tips of the thumb and little finger touch.

C

Cannon Breath

Relates to the breath of fire, but here the breath is through the mouth. Also used as a final, powerful exhale at the end of an exercise.

Celibate Pose

Seated pose in which the seat is placed on the floor between the kneeling legs.

Chakra (= wheel, disk, circle)

Psychoenergetic energy fields along the spine.

D

Dharana

Sixth level of eight-limbed yoga: concentration.

Dhyana

Seventh level of eight-limbed yoga: meditation.

G

Gatka

Sword martial art of the Sikhs; also indicates the staff dancing which developed from it.

Gurmukhi

The holy language of the Sikhs, related to Sanskrit.

Guru (gu = dark; ru = light)

Brings emotional and spiritual growth and shares knowledge; this can occur through people as well as through duties, situations, or books.

Gyan (Jnana) Yoga (= the path of knowledge)

One of the four classical yoga paths with the goal of arriving at the release from the cycle of reincarnation through study.

Gyan Mudra

Seal of wisdom; hand position in which the tips of the thumb and index finger touch.

H

Half Lotus Position

Simplified lotus position, in which just one foot is laid over the opposite thigh.

Hatha Yoga (ha = sun; tha = moon)

The path of body awareness; the most well-known form of yoga in the West, with an emphasis on physical exercises/the physical aspects.

Hatha Yoga Pradipika

A well-known yoga text from the fifteenth century; describes the difference between Hatha and Raja Yoga.

I

Ida
Energy channel for distribution of apana.

J

Jalandhara Bandha
Throat lock; lengthening of the neck and engaging of the neck musculature.

K

Karma Yoga (= the path of selfless service)
One of the four classical yoga paths with the goal of using up existing karma.

Kriya (= position)
A specific exercise series. Can also be a single, standalone exercise.

Kundalini (= serpent energy)
The highest spiritual power in humans.

L

Lion Breath
Powerful mouth breath with a stuck out tongue.

Long Deep Breath
Yogic breath/basic breath method in yoga; has a calming and cooling effect.

Lotus Position
Classic seated pose for meditation, in which the tops of the feet are laid on the opposite thighs.

M

Maha Bandha (= great seal)
Simultaneously engaging mula bandha, uddhyana bandha, and jalandhara bandha.

Mantra (= projection of the mind)
Sound formulas as tools for concentration and meditation.

Meridian
Energy paths in the body (according to the teachings of traditional Chinese medicine).

Mudra
Hand and finger positions, through which body energy is stimulated and channeled.

Mula Bandha
Root lock; locking the three lower chakras.

N

Nadi
Subtle body energy paths in the body for distributing prana; comparable to the meridians in traditional Chinese medicine.

Nadi Sodhana
    Breathing alternately through the left and right nostril.

Niyama
    Second level of eight-limbed yoga: self-discipline.

P

Patanjali
    Indian yogi and philosopher (ca. 2 B.C.E.); supposed writer of the *Yoga Sutras*.

Pingala
    Energy channel for distributing prana.

Prana (= life breath, life power, energy, air)
    Universal life energy.

Pranam Mudra
    Prayer position; hand position, in which the palms are placed together in front of the chest.

Pranayama
    Fourth level of eight-limbed yoga: breath control.

Pratyahara
    Fifth level of eight-limbed yoga: control of the senses.

R

Raya Yoga (= the royal path)
    One of the four classical yoga paths with the goal of controlling the mind. KUNDALINI YOGA is a Raya Yoga.

S

Sadhana
    Daily, spiritual practice.

Samadhi
    Eighth level of eight-limbed yoga: enlightenment.

Samyama
    Umbrella term for the last three meditative levels of ashtanga: dharana, dhyana, and samadhi.

Sanskrit
    The oldest Indian language; still the holy language and scholarly language of Hindu.

Sat Kriya
    An exercise in KUNDALINI YOGA.

SAT NAM (sat = truth; nam = identity)
    Most commonly used mantra; always sung at the end of a yoga practice session.

Sat Nam Rasayan (= the essence of the true being)
    Meditative-spiritual healing technique from the tradition of KUNDALINI YOGA, passed on by Yogi Bhajan.

Shakti (= strength)
    Female principle of creation; the dynamic, creative energy.

Shiva (= the gracious)
    Male principle of creation; the still, observant energy.

Shuni Mudra
Seal of patience; hand position in which the tips of the thumb and middle finger touch.

Simple Seated Pose
Also called simple pose; the most common seated pose in KUNDALINI YOGA, in which the legs are crossed and the heels are brought as close as possible to the pelvis.

Sitali Pranayama
Cooling breath through the rolled tongue.

Solar Plexus
Corresponds to the navel chakra.

Surya Mudra
Seal of the sun; hand position in which the tips of the thumb and ring finger touch.

Sushmana (also called sushumna)
The main energy channel in the body, along the spine.

T

Third Eye
Sixth chakra; concentration point between the eyebrows.

U

Uddhyana Bandha
Diaphragm lock: engaging the upper stomach and the diaphragm.

V

Venus Lock
Hand position in which the fingers are intertwined.

Y

Yama
First level of eight-limbed yoga: abstinence, self-control.

Yoga (= yoke, binding)
Term for the connection of body, mind, and soul.

Yoga Sutra (= yoga guide)
Describes the essence of yoga in short, reduced verse form.

Yogi Bhajan
Master of KUNDALINI YOGA; spread this yoga technique in the Western world.

3HO
Healthy Happy Holy Organization, founded in 1969 by Yogi Bhajan.

REFERENCES

KRIYAS

Page 106 Sat Kriya: Sadhana Handbuch, KRI, first English edition 1974
Page 108 Varuyas Kriya: Sadhana Handbuch, KRI, first English edition 1974
Page 110 Wake-Up Series: Relax and Renew*
Page 112 Awakening the Kundalini Energy: Relax and Renew*
Page 114 Basic Spinal Energy Series: Sadhana Handbuch, KRI, first English edition 1974
Page 116 Kriya for Strengthening Disease Resistance: Keeping up with Kundalini Yoga, KRI 1980
Page 118 Kriya for Overcoming Insomnia: Sadhana Handbuch, KRI, first English edition 1974
Page 120 Exercise Series for the Kidneys: The Aquarian Teacher, Level 1, KRI 2003
Page 122 New Opportunities and Green Energy: Relax and Renew*
Page 126 Cleansing Series for Beginners: Sadhana Handbuch, KRI, first English edition 1974
Page 128 Surya Kriya: Sadhana Handbuch, KRI, first English edition 1974
Page 130 Give Your Liver Strength: Owner's Manual for the Human Body, Yogi Bhajan, 1993
Page 132 Nabhi Kriya: Kundalini Meditation Manual for Intermediate Students, KRI 1977
Page 134 Kriya for Purification of the Self: Sadhana Handbuch, KRI, first English edition 1974
Page 136 Kriya for Pelvic Balance: Keeping up with Kundalini Yoga, KRI 1980
Page 138 Coordinating Body, Mind, and Soul: Self Knowledge, Yogi Bhajan 1995
Page 140 Meditation and Self-Reliance: Kundalini Meditation Manual for Intermediate Students,
       KRI 1977

*The guide to this kriya is taken from Gururattan Kaur Khalsas's Relax and Renew and thus could not be verified for authenticity and accuracy by the Kundalini Research Institute.

MEDITATION

Quote on page 145 from Kundalini Yoga, German Teacher Training Level 1, basic course 1, p. 2 (Quote originally from Naranjo & Ornstein)

Page 146 Seven Wave SAT NAME Meditation: Sadhana Handbuch, KRI, first English edition 1974
Page 148 Emotional Balance: German Teacher Training Level 1
Page 151 Concentration in Action: Survival Kit, Yogi Bhajan, 1980
Page 152 Meditation to Free Yourself from Depression: The Aquarian Teacher, Stufe 1, KRI 2003
Page 155 Meditation Against Addictive Habits: Kundalini Yoga as Taught by Yogi Bhajan, Shakta
       Kaur Khalsa, Dorling Kindersley 2001
Page 156 Kirtan Kriya: Sadhana Handbuch, KRI, first English edition 1974
Page 158 Beggar's Meditation: Kundalini Meditation Manual for Intermediate Students, KRI 1977
Page 160 Kriya of the Smiling Buddha: Kundalini Meditation Manual for Intermediate Students,
       KRI 1977
Page 162 Ungali Pranayama: Kundalini Meditation Manual for Intermediate Students, KRI 1977
Page 164 Healing: Transitions to a Heart-Centered World** and The Aquarian Teacher, Stufe 1,
       KRI 2003
Page 167 Meditation for Change: Kundalini Meditation Manual for Intermediate Students, KRI 1977
Page 168 Meditation for Self-Assessment: Kundalini Meditation Manual for Intermediate Students,
       KRI 1977

** The guide to this meditation is taken from Gururattan Kaur Khalsas's book Transitions to a Heart-Centered World and thus could not be verified for authenticity and accuracy by the Kundalini Research Institute.

MANTRA

Page 171 The notation for "Long Time Sun …" was taken from the book Kundalini Yoga as Taught by Yogi Bhajan by Shakta Kaur Khalsa, Dorling Kindersley 2001.

BIBLIOGRAPHY

3HO Deutschland: Handbuch für Lehrer und Studenten

Anand Kaur Seitz: Kundalini Yoga, Harmonie für Körper und Seele durch die Chakra-Energien,
Rowohlt Taschenbuch Verlag, Hamburg 1999

Andrea Christiansen: Mudras, Fingeryoga für mehr Wohlbefinden und Lebensfreude,
Südwest Verlag, München 2005

Cai Pfannstiel: Handbuch Yoga, Grundlagen, Übungen und Techniken,
Deutscher Taschenbuchverlag, München 1997

Dr. Wulf Splitstoeßer: Die Unterweisungen des Yoghi Bajan, Ph.D., Die Macht des gesprochenen Wortes,
Dr. Splitstoeßer Verlag, Kelkheim 2004

Genevieve Lewis Paulson: Kundalini and the Chakras,
Rootlight, Levelyn Publications, St.Paul/USA 2003

Gururattan Kaur Khalsa: Relax and Renew,
Yoga Technology Press, San Diego/USA 1988

Gururattan Kaur Khalsa: Transitions to a heart-centered world,
Yoga Technology Press, San Diego/USA 1988

Owner´s Manual for the Human Body, Yogi Bhajan, 1993
Joseph Michael Levry (Gurunam): Den Schleier lüften, Praktische Kabbalah mit Kundalini Yoga,
Rootlight, New York/USA, dt. Ausgabe 2004

KUNDALINI YOGA Lehrerausbildung Stufe I

Paramhans Swami Maheshwarananda: Die verborgenen Kräfte im Menschen, Chakras und Kundalini,
Ibera Verlag/European University Press, Wien 2002

Rajah von Aundh: Das Sonnengebet, Ein einfaches System von Yoga-Übungen für Jedermann,
Artha Verlag, Haslach 1997

Sadhana Handbuch, KRI, first English edition 1974

Satya Singh: Das Kundalini Yoga Handbuch, für Gesundheit von Körper, Geist und Seele,
Wilhelm Heyne Verlag, München 2003

Shakta Kaur Khalsa: Kundalini Yoga as taught by Yogi Bhajan,
Dorling Kindersley, New York/USA 2001

Shakti Parwha Kaur Khalsa: Kundalini Yoga,
The Flow of Eternal Power, Perigee, New York/USA 1996

Sukadev V Bretz: Das Yoga Vidya Asana Buch. Yogareihen,
basierend auf der Rishikeshreihe nach Swami Sivananda,
Yoga Vidya Verlag, Frankfurt

Yogi Bhajan, The Aquarian Teacher,
KRI International Kundalini Yoga Teacher Training, 2003

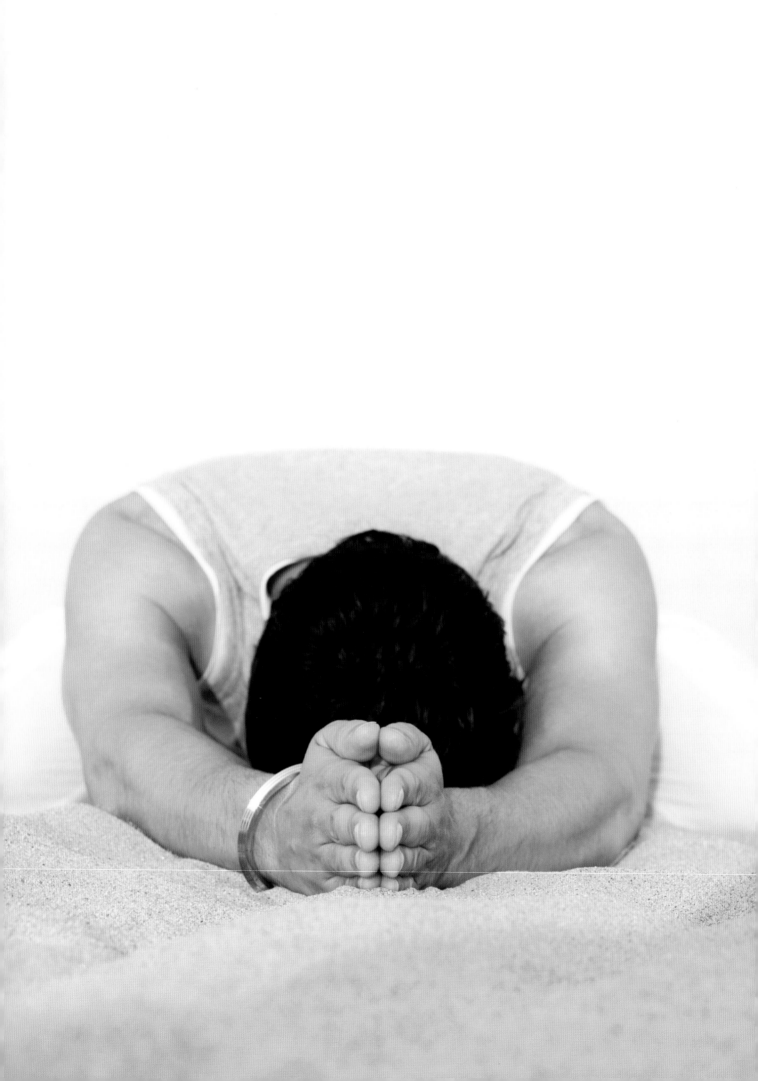

ACKNOWLEDGMENTS

Dear Brigitte, I would like to first give you my special and heartfelt thanks. Without your wonderful photographs and your support, this book would never have come to be. Your belief in us and our idea helped me to realize this project. Many thanks for your commitment to our work, from the giant photo selection and editing to your support with formulating the text and your suggestions for improvement. I thank you for our wonderful friendship, mutual trust, your wealth of ideas, and your motivating energy. This book is inseparably connected to you.

I thank Julian Rupp for assistance with photo production, edition, and for the limitless and universal commitment during the entire project. Thank you for your enriching corrections, recommendations, and knowledge of wording.

I thank Claudia Rendenbach for her patient work on the redrafting and editing of the entire test. Thank you for the understanding, the dedication, and the cooperation.

I would like the thank Annette Hodge for being ready to work with me as a model. Thank you for the great time together in Greece and for the beautiful performances.

Siri Kauer Magerfleisch also deserves my thanks for the many constructive suggestions and bringing in her knowledge of yoga. Thank you for your patience with the correction of the text.

I owe great thanks to Angela Thomaschik and Heike Heckl from Umchau Publishing for their interest in the book and the topic. Thank you for the successful, harmonic cooperation.

I thank Ines Siri Tapa Kaur Driebe immensely for her dynamic support through the entire project.

I thank Federico Orozco for taking me to my very first yoga class. Thank you for all the steps we have taken and experiences we have had together on the yoga path.

A hearty thanks goes to Hari Dev Kaur and Jagat Kaur for the many intensive weekends in Spain. Thank you for the realization that yoga is not just exercise, but a life path.

My deep, heartfelt thanks goes to my parents for their unconditional love. Thank you for the infinite support for all my decisions, plans, and in all circumstances. A big thanks for the support and accommodation for a part of the photo production in Greece.

I thank my sister Theonitsa and her husband Stephan Zoller for their love, understanding, and moral, powerful, and energetic support. Thank you for believing in this project.

My thanks also goes to Yogi Bhajan for his decision to teach KUNDALINI YOGA openly in the West, giving us all the chance to encounter this philosophy. Thank you for changing and enriching my life in wonderful ways through KUNDALINI YOGA.

With love and gratitude,
Sat Nam,
Athanasios Karta Singh

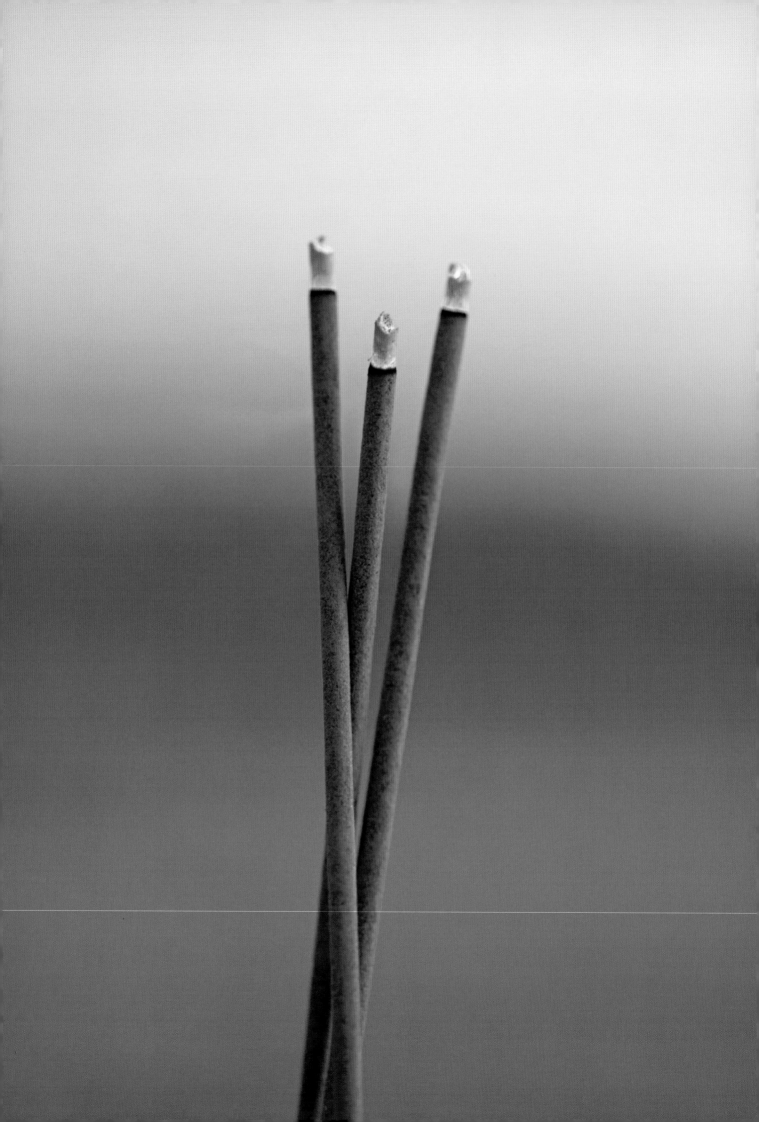

MAY THE LONG TIME SUN
SHINE UPON YOU
ALL LOVE SURROUND YOU
AND THE PURE LIGHT WITHIN YOU
GUIDE YOUR WAY ON

SAT NAM

CREDITS

Text
Athanasios Karta Singh Megarisiotis, Munich

Photography
Brigitte Sporrer, Munich

Portrait Photography
Julian Rupp

Photograph of Yogi Bhajan, page 15, used with the kind approval of the Kundalini Research Institute.

KRI Approval
Siri Kaur Magerfleisch, Hamburg

Layout
Athanasios Karta Singh Megarisiotis, Munich

Typesetting and Design
Tischewski & Tischewski, Marburg

Editor and Project Management
Angela Thomaschik, Neustadt/Weinstraße

Production
Heike Heckl, Neustadt/Weinstraße

Reproduction
RGD, Digitale Medientechnik, Langen